Radiological English

R. Ribes · P. R. Ros

Ramón Ribes · Pablo R. Ros

Radiological English

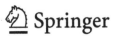 Springer

Ramón Ribes, MD, PhD
Hospital Reina Sofia
Servicio de Radiología
Avda. Menéndez Pidal s/n.
Córdoba 14004, Spain

Pablo R. Ros, MD, MPH
Professor of Radiology, Harvard Medical School
Executive Vice Chairman and Associate Radiologist-in-Chief,
Brigham and Women's Hospital
Chief, Division of Radiology, Dana-Farber Cancer Institute
Harvard Medical School
75 Francis St.
Boston, MA 02115, USA

ISBN-10   3-540-29328-0 Springer Berlin Heidelberg New York
ISBN-13   978-3-540-29328-6 Springer Berlin Heidelberg New York

Library of Congress Control Number: 2006929202

Springer is a part of Springer Science+Business Media

springer.com

© Springer-Verlag Berlin · Heidelberg 2007

Editor: Dr. Ute Heilmann, Springer-Verlag
Desk Editor: Wilma McHugh, Springer-Verlag
Production: LE-TEX Jelonek, Schmidt & Vöckler GbR, Leipzig
Typesetting: K+V Fotosatz GmbH, Beerfelden
Cover design: Estudio Calamar, F. Steinen-Broo, Pau/Girona, Spain

24/3100/YL – 5 4 3 2 1 0 – Printed on acid-free paper

To Rosario Alarcon, I do admire you as my wife, as the mother of my two daughters and as a successful professional.

R. Ribes

To Silvia, my wife.

P. R. Ros

Preface

For all of us non-native English speakers, to learn English has been a challenge at a certain point in our lives. Furthermore, we would guess that none of us in the healthcare profession has had much training in medical English or, more specifically, radiological English. It is said that theologians, lawyers, engineers and physicians speak in a different language from the rest of society; for us who practice the radiological sciences, the learning of radiological English has typically been a "learn on the job" experience.

Radiological English is by far the most demanding medical specialty English since radiologists need to know not only radiological terminology, but also that of referring physicians. In the years of residency before becoming involved in a particular subspecialty, radiology residents talk to virtually all specialists in the hospital, so they are exposed to a great deal of medical terminology which at the beginning seems impossible to manage.

Probably that was the reason why we began to write *Medical English* which was also published by Springer. Although writing *Medical English* required a great deal of time and effort, we believe it was easier for us as radiologists than for any other specialist. This may explain the scarcity of books teaching medical English written by doctors.

After having written a book on general medical English, we felt the pressing need to write a second book on the medical English we talk on a daily basis and are interested in: radiological English. From the beginning we realized that even within radiology there are many kinds of spoken (and heard) radiological English.

In this book we have tried to be as comprehensive as possible, so it is divided into units containing different aspects of communication in radiological English. After an introductory unit on the method of approaching radiological English, we touch upon specific radiological grammar, scientific literature and how to write letters to radiological journals. We have also included units on tips to attend international courses on radiology and specifically on giving a radiology talk or chairing a scientific session. There are also units on how to use Latin and Greek terms in medical English including singular and plural forms. We close the first portion of the book with the most common dreaded acronyms and abbreviations used by radiologists who are native English speakers.

The second portion of the book refers to radiology reporting with units dealing with describing lesions and composing reports, both normal and abnormal. The third portion of the book deals with "dialects" in radiological English. English speakers are fascinated with different forms of speaking English in different parts of the world such as the United States, Ireland or New Zealand. The same happens in radiology where there are some specific "dialects" of radiological English in: (1) interventional radiology, (2) on call where a lot of slang terms are used and, finally, (3) in radiological management where administrators use a number of key terms that permeate the specialty. We close the book with three units on conversational radiological English, communication skills in medicine and a survival conversation guide.

We really hope this book will be helpful to professionals working within the realm of radiology who are non-native English speakers. This would include not only radiologists, either trained or in training, but also technologists, nurses, administrators, basic scientists, and others who work in diagnostic imaging and its subspecialties. We had fun putting together this book, thinking about areas to cover and enlisting collaborators who like us were interested in the subtleties of communication in radiology at many levels. But now, the final test rests in you the reader. We are sure that you will find situations that will appear familiar to you, and the book will be helpful in improving your communication skills in this specialty based so much on communication with patients, referring physicians and other radiological professionals. Please let us know how to improve this book and send us your experiences so we can start working on a second edition of *Radiological English.*

In short, this manual is intended to make the adaptation to an English-speaking radiological environment easier for you than it was for us since there is no time to be wasted when you are faced with such a great opportunity of personal and radiological development. We hope you enjoy reading this manual as much as we have enjoyed writing it.

Ramón Ribes, MD, PhD
Pablo R. Ros, MD, MPH, FACR

Acknowledgements

We would like to thank Hansel Otero, MD, for his valuable help in the preparation of Unit XVI.

We would like to thank Mildred Dewire for her assistance in preparing the manuscript.

Contents

Unit IV
Letters to Editors of Radiological Journals

Unit V
Attending an International Radiological Course

Unit VI
Giving a Radiological Talk

Unit VII
Chairing a Radiological Session

Unit VIII
Usual Mistakes Made by Radiologists Speaking and Writing in English

Unit IX
Latin and Greek Terminology

Unit X
Acronyms and Abbreviations

Unit XI
Describing a Lesion

Unit XII
Standard Normal Reports

Unit XIII
Reporting in English

Unit XIV
Interventional Radiology

Unit XV
On Call

Unit XVI
Radiological Management

Unit XVII
Radiological Conversation Guide

Unit XVIII
Basic Communication Skills in Medicine

Unit XIX
Conversation Survival Guide

Contributors

Bang Huynh
Radiology resident at Brigham
and Women's Hospital
Boston, MA, USA
Contributed to the preparation
of Units V, VIII, XII, XIII, XIV, XV,
XVII, and XVIII

José Luis Sancho
Radiologist at Alto Guadalquivir
Hospital
Andújar (Jaén), Spain
Contributed to the preparation
of Units II, III, V, XI, XII, XIII,
and XIX

José María Vida
Radiologist at Montilla Hospital
Montilla (Córdoba), Spain
Contributed to the preparation
of Units VI, VIII, IX, and X

José María Martos
Radiology resident at Reina Sofía
Hospital
Cordoba, Spain
Contributed to the preparation
of Units II, III, and V

Rocío Díaz
Radiology resident at Reina Sofía
Hospital
Córdoba, Spain
Contributed to the preparation
of Units IX, X, and XVII

Eloisa Feliú
Radiologist at INSCANNER
Alicante, Spain
Contributed to the preparation
of Unit III

Silvia Ondategui-Parra,
MD, MPH, MSc
Administration Dana Farber Cancer
Institute
Brigham and Women's Hospital
Harvard Medical School
Boston, MA, USA
Contributed to the preparation
of Unit XVI

Antonio Luna
Radiologist at Clínica Las Nieves
Jaén, Spain
Contributed to the preparation
of Unit IV

Pedro Aranda
Cardiovascular Surgeon at Carlos
Haya Hospital
Málaga, Spain
Contributed to the preparation
of Unit XVIII

Francisco Muñoz del Castillo
Family doctor and ENT Consultant
at Reina Sofía Hospital
Córdoba, Spain
Drew the cartoons

UNIT I

Unit I   Methodological Approach to Radiological English

Introduction

The learning of radiological English is probably the most demanding of all medical English by specialty. On the one hand, radiology covers the whole anatomy, physiology and pathology of the body, so radiologists in the years of residency, before getting involved in a radiological subspecialty, must be familiar with virtually all medical English terminology; there is no other specialty in which this happens. Cardiologists are not interested at all in meniscal tears and orthopedic surgeons do not need to know a word about arrhythmias (not even arrhythmia itself, which is one of the most frequently misspelled medical words). On the other hand, the multiplicity of radiological subspecialties makes it extremely difficult, even for radiologists, to be familiar with the jargon of each subspecialty: an interventional radiologist would be completely lost in a talk on mammography, and a mammographer might not know the name of most interventional radiology devices.

A sound knowledge of English grammar is pivotal in order to build your radiological English consistently. To be fluent in anatomical English is crucial for radiologists; we need to know what the normal structures look like and are called, and how to express their relationships with radiological findings. Anatomy is so linked to Latin and Greek that unless you are familiar with Latin and Greek terminology you will never be able to speak and write either anatomical or radiological English properly. Besides, radiologists must be aware of the technical aspects of their subspecialties and must be able to talk about them in an intelligible manner to patients, referring physicians, residents, nurses, and technicians.

Besides the technical medical language, the radiologist must understand patients' medical English which is the language used by patients talking about their conditions. Both in ultrasound and interventional radiology, patients talk about their conditions to the radiologists, but don't forget than in CT and MR units patients are interviewed by technologists who must be aware of the usual expressions used by patients with regard to their illnesses.

Let's do a simple exercise. Read this sentence of radiological English:

1) Furthermore, ghost image artifacts arising from the intraluminal signal can be used to prove the vascular nature of these lesions.

We are sure you understand the sentence and that you are able to translate it into your own language almost instantly; unfortunately translation is not only useless but deleterious to your radiological English with regard to fluency.

If you try to read the paragraph in English out-loud, your first difficulties will appear.

If a conversation on the sentence starts and the audience is waiting for your opinion, you may begin to sweat.

If you are not currently doing MR, "ghost artifact" (*UK*: artefact) may mean nothing to you.

Check the words you are not able to pronounce easily and look them up in the dictionary.

Ask an English-speaking colleague to read it aloud; try to write it; probably you will find some difficulty in writing certain words.

Check the words you are not able to write properly and look them up in the dictionary.

Finally, try to have a conversation on the topic.

Notice how many problems have been raised by just one sentence of radiological English. Our advice is that once you have diagnosed your actual radiological English level:

Do not get depressed if it is below your expectations.

Keep doing these exercises with progressively longer paragraphs beginning with those belonging to your subspecialty.

Arrange radiological English sessions at your institution. A session once a week might be a good starting point. The sessions will keep you, and your colleagues, in touch with at least a weekly radiological English meeting. You will notice that you feel much more confident talking to colleagues with a lower level than yours than talking to your native English teacher as you will feel better talking to non-native English-speaking radiologists than talking to native English-speaking colleagues. In these sessions you can rehearse the performance of talks and lectures so that when you give a presentation at an international meeting it is not the first time it has been delivered.

Let's evaluate our radiological English level with these ten simple (?) exercises:

Are the following five sentences correct?

1. Baker's cysts are hyperintense on T2.
   – NOT CORRECT

The use of "-weighted image" after T1, T2, and PD is imperative since all images contain T1, T2, and PD information, and we call sequences with regard to their predominant, although not exclusive, weighting. Therefore the correct sentence is:

- Baker's cysts are hyperintense on T2-weighted images.

2. The flexor digitorum long tendon is rarely involved with abnormalities.
   – NOT CORRECT

The correct sentence is:

- The flexor digitorum longus tendon is rarely involved with abnormalities.

Always double-check Latin/Greek terminology spellings.

3. 57-years-old patient with severe abdominal pain.
   – NOT CORRECT

The correct sentence is:

- 57-year-old patient with severe abdominal pain.

"57-year-old" is, in this case, an adjective, and adjectives, when they precede a name, cannot be written in the plural.

4. There was not biopsy of the lesion.
   – NOT CORRECT

The correct sentence is:

- There was no biopsy of the lesion.

We could have said instead "there was not a biopsy of the lesion" or "there was not any biopsy of the lesion".

5. 87-year-old patient with arrythmia.
   – NOT CORRECT

"Arrhythmia" is one of the most commonly misspelled words in medical English. You can avoid this recurrent mistake by checking that the word "rhythm" (provided it is spelled correctly!) is embedded in "arrhythmia".

6. What does "window an image" mean?

To adjust the appropriate window and level settings.

7. What would you understand if in an interventional radiology suite you hear: "Dance with me"?

Someone is asking to have his/her gown tied up.

8. Are "Harvard students" and "Harvard alumni" synonymous?

NO. The former term refers to current students and the latter to former students.

9. How would you ask a patient to perform a Valsalva maneuver?

Bear down as if you are having a bowel movement.

10. Are "home calls" and "in-house calls" synonymous?

NO. They are not synonymous but antonymous; they express opposite concepts. In "home calls" you will hopefully sleep at home, whereas in "in-house calls" you must stay in the hospital for the whole clinical duty.

This set of questions is intended for those who think that radiological English is not worth giving a second thought to. On the one hand, most radiologists who have never worked in English-speaking hospitals tend to underestimate the difficulty of radiological English; they think that provided you speak English you will not find any problems in radiological environments. On the other hand, those who have suffered in their own skins embarrassing situations working abroad, do not dare say that either English or radiological English are easy.

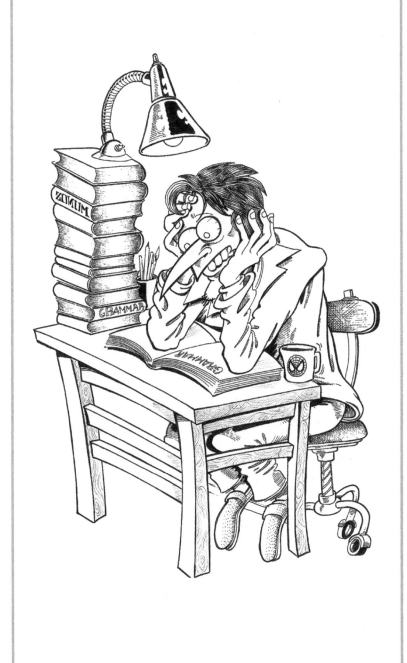

Unit II Radiological Grammar

The first chapters are probably the least read by most readers in general and radiologists in particular, and in our opinion it is precisely in the first chapters that the most important information of a book is displayed. It is in its first chapters that the foundations of a book are laid, and many readers do not optimize the reading of a manual because they skip its fundamentals.

This is a vital chapter because unless you have a sound knowledge of English grammar you will be absolutely unable to speak English as is expected from a well-trained radiologist. At your expected English level it is definitely not enough just to be understood; you must speak fluently and your command of the English language must allow you to communicate with your colleagues regardless of their nationality.

As you will see immediately, this grammar section is made up of radiological sentences, so at the same time that you revise, for instance, the passive voice, you will be reviewing how to say usual sentences in day-to-day radiological English such as "the CT scan had already been performed when the Chairman arrived at the CT Unit".

We could say, to summarize, that we have replaced the classical sentence of old English manuals "my tailor is rich" by expressions such as "the first year radiology resident is on call today". Without a certain grammatical background it is not possible to speak correctly just as without a certain knowledge of anatomy it would not be possible to report on radiological examinations. The tendency to skip both grammar and anatomy, considered by many as simple preliminary issues, has had deleterious effects on the learning of English and radiology.

Tenses

Talking About the Present

Present continuous

Present continuous shows an action that is happening in the present time at or around the moment of speaking.

Present simple of the verb *to be* + gerund of the verb: *am/are/is* ...-ing. Study this example:

- It is 7.30 in the morning. Dr. Hudson is in his new car on his way to the Radiology Department.

So: He *is driving* to the radiology department. He is driving to the radiology department means that he is driving now, at the time of speaking.

USES

To talk about:

- Something that is happening at the time of speaking (i.e., now):
  - Dr. Hudson *is going* to the fluoroscopy room.
  - Dr. Smith's colleague *is performing* an enteroclysis.

- Something that is happening around or close to the time of speaking, but not necessarily exactly at the time of speaking:
  - Jim and John are residents of radiology and they are having a sandwich in the cafeteria. John says: "I *am writing* an interesting article on double-contrast barium enema. I'll lend it to you when I've finished it". As you can see John is not writing the article at the time of speaking. He means that he has begun to write the article but has not finished it yet. He is in the middle of writing it.

- Something that is happening for a limited period of time around the present (e.g., today, this week, this season, this year ...):
  - Our junior radiology residents *are working* hard this term.

- Changing situations:
  - Radiologically speaking, the patient's condition *is getting* better.

- Temporary situations:
  - I *am living* with other residents until I can buy my own apartment.
  - I *am doing* a rotation in the MR division until the end of May.

Special use: Present continuous with a future meaning
In the following examples doing these things is already arranged.

- To talk about what you have arranged to do in the near future (personal arrangements).
  - We *are stenting* a renal artery on Monday.
  - I *am having* dinner with an interventional radiologist from the United States tomorrow.

We can also use the form *going to* in these sentences, but it is less natural when you talk about arrangements.
We do not use the simple present or *will* for personal arrangements.

Simple present

Simple present shows an action that happens again and again (repeated action) in the present time, but not necessarily at the time of speaking.

<table>
<tr>
<td>FORM</td>
<td>

The simple present has the following forms:

- Affirmative (remember to add -s or -es to the third person singular)

- Negative
  - I/we/you/they don't ...
  - He/she/it doesn't ...

- Interrogative
  - Do I/we/you/they ...?
  - Does he/she/it ...?
  Study this example:

- Dr. Allan is the chairman of the Radiology Department. He is at an international course in Greece at this moment.
  So: He *is not running* the Radiology Department now (because he is in Greece), but *he runs* the Radiology Department.

</td>
</tr>
</table>

<table>
<tr>
<td>USES</td>
<td>

- To talk about something that happens all the time or repeatedly or something that is true in general. Here it is not important whether the action is happening at the time of speaking:
  - I *do* interventional radiology.
  - Nurses *take care* of patients after an angiography procedure.
  - For GI exams, pre-examination preparation *serves* to cleanse the bowel.

- To say how often we do things:
  - I *begin* to dictate studies at 8.30 every morning.
  - Dr. Taylor *does* angioplasty two evenings a week.
  - How often *do you go* to an international radiology course? Once a year.

- For a permanent situation (a situation that stays the same for a long time):
  - I *work* as a mammographer in the breast cancer program of our hospital. I have been working there for ten years.

- Some verbs are used only in simple tenses. These verbs are verbs of thinking or mental activity, feeling, possession and perception, and reporting verbs. We often use *can* instead of the present tense with verbs of perception:

</td>
</tr>
</table>

USES

- I *can understand* now why the X-ray machine is in such a bad condition.
- I *can see* now the solution to the diagnostic problem.

● The simple present is often used with adverbs of frequency such as *always, often, sometimes, rarely, never, every week*, and *twice a year*:
  - The radiology chairman *always* works very hard.
  - We *have* a radiology conference *every week*.

● Simple present with a future meaning. We use it to talk about timetables, schedules ...:
  - What time *does* the radiation safety conference *start*? It *starts* at 9.30.

Talking About the Future

Going To

USES

● To say what we have already decided to do or what we intend to do in the future (do not use *will* in this situation):
  - I *am going to* attend the 20th International Congress of Radiology next month.
  - There is a CT course in Boston next fall. *Are you going to* attend it?

● To say what someone has arranged to do (personal arrangements), but remember that we prefer to use the present continuous because it sounds more natural:
  - What time *are you going to meet* the vice chairman?
  - What time *are you going to* begin the angiogram?

● To say what we think will happen (making predictions):
  - The patient is agitated. I think we *are not going to* get a good quality study.
  - *Oh, the patient's* chest X-ray looks terrible. "I think he is going to die soon" the radiologist said.

● If we want to say what someone intended to do in the past but did not do, we use *was/were going to*:
  - He *was going to* do a CT on the patient but finally changed his mind and decided to do an MR.

● To talk about past predictions we use *was/were going to*:
  - The resident had the feeling that the patient *was going to* suffer a reaction to the contrast material.

Simple Future (Will)

FORM	I/We *will* or *shall* (*will* is more common than *shall. Shall* is often used in questions to make offers and suggestions): • *Shall* we go to the contrast media symposium next week? Oh, great idea! *You/he/she/it/they will.* Negative: *shan't, won't.*

USES	• We use *will* when we decide to do something at the time of speaking (remember that in this situation, you cannot use the simple present): – Have you finished the report? – No, I haven't had time to do it. – OK, don't worry, I *will* do it. • When offering, agreeing, refusing and promising to do something, or when asking someone to do something: – That case looks difficult for you. Do not worry, I **will** help you out. – Can I have the book about high-resolution of the lung that I lent you back? Of course. I *will* give it back to you tomorrow. – Don't ask to perform the ultrasound examination by yourself. The consultant *won't* allow you to. – I promise I *will* send you a copy of the latest article on ultrasound-guided biopsy as soon as I get it. – *Will* you help me out with this cystogram, please? You do not use *will* to say what someone has already decided to do or arranged to do (remember that in this situation we use *going to* or the present continuous). • To predict a future happening or a future situation: – The specialty of radiology *will* be very different in a hundred years' time. – Chest MRI *won't* be the same in the next two decades. Remember that if there is something in the present situation that shows us what will happen in the future (near future) we use *going to* instead of *will.* • With expressions such as: *probably, I am sure, I bet, I think, I suppose, I guess*: – I *will probably* attend the European Congress.

USES	– You should listen to Dr. Helms giving a conference. I am *sure* you *will* love it. – I *bet* the patient *will* recover satisfactorily after the reaction following the administration of contrast material. – I *guess* I *will* see you at the next annual meeting.

Future Continuous

FORM	*Will be* + gerund of the verb.

USES	• To say that we will be in the middle of something at a certain time in the future: – This time tomorrow morning I *will be performing* my first myelogram. • To talk about things that are already planned or decided (similar to the present continuous with a future meaning): – We can't meet this evening. I *will be stenting the aneurysm* in the patient we talked about. • To ask about people's plans, especially when we want something or want someone to do something (interrogative form): – *Will* you *be helping* me dictate MR reports this evening?

Future Perfect

FORM	*Will have* + past participle of the verb. • To say that something will already have happened before a certain time in the future: – I think the resident *will* already *have arrived* by the time we begin the scrotal ultrasound. – Next spring I *will have been working* for 25 years in the Radiology Department of this institution.

Talking About the Past

Simple Past

<table>
<tr>
<td>FORM</td>
<td>

The simple past has the following forms:

- Affirmative:
  - The past of the regular verbs is formed by adding -ed to the infinitive.
  - The past of the irregular verbs has its own form.

- Negative:
  - Did/didn't + the base form of the verb.

- Questions:
  - Did I/you/ ... + the base form of the verb.

</td>
</tr>
</table>

<table>
<tr>
<td>USES</td>
<td>

- To talk about actions or situations in the past (they have already finished):
  - I really enjoyed the radiology residents' party very much.
  - When I worked as a visiting resident in Madrid, I performed one hundred stereotactically guided core biopsies.

- To say that one thing happened after another:
  - Yesterday we had a terrible duty. We did a carotid angiogram in five patients and then we performed an aneurysm embolization.

- To ask or say when or what time something happened:
  - When were you last on call?

- To tell a story and to talk about happenings and actions that are not connected with the present (historical events):
  - Roentgen discovered X-rays.

</td>
</tr>
</table>

Past Continuous

<table>
<tr>
<td>FORM</td>
<td>Was/were + gerund of the verb.</td>
</tr>
</table>

USES

- To say that someone was in the middle of doing something at a certain time. The action or situation had already started before this time but hadn't finished:

- This time last year I *was writing* the article on contrast-enhanced MRI features of ankylosing spondylitis that has been recently published.

Notice that the past continuous does not tell us whether an action was finished or not. Perhaps it was, perhaps it was not.

- To describe a scene:
  – A lot of patients *were waiting* in the corridor to have their chest X-ray done.

Present Perfect

FORM

Have/has + past participle of the verb.

USES

- To talk about the present result of a past action.
- To talk about a recent happening.

In the latter situation you can use the present perfect with the following particles:

- *Just* (i.e., a short time ago): to say something has happened a short time ago:
  – Dr. Ho *has just arrived* at the hospital. He is our new pediatric radiologist.
- *Already*: to say something has happened sooner than expected:
  – The second-year resident *has already finished* her presentation.

Remember that to talk about a recent happening we can also use the simple past:

- To talk about a period of time that continues up to the present (an unfinished period of time):
  – We use the expressions: *today, this morning, this evening, this week* ...
  – We often use *ever* and *never*.
- To talk about something that we are expecting. In this situation we use *yet* to show that the speaker is expecting something to happen, but only in questions and negative sentences:

– Dr. Helms *has not arrived yet.*

- To talk about something you have never done or something you have not done during a period of time that continues up to the present:
  – I *have not reported* an MR scan of the knee since I was a resident.

- To talk about how much we have done, how many things we have done or how many times we have done something:
  – I *have reported* that regional brain perfusion scan twice because the first report was lost.
  – Dr. Yimou *has performed* twenty vertebroplasties this week.

- To talk about situations that exist for a long time, especially if we say *always.* In this case the situation still exists now:
  – Gadolinium *has always been* the contrast agent used in MRI examinations.
  – Dr. Olmedo *has always been* a very talented radiologist.

We also use the present perfect with these expressions:

- Superlative: *It is the most ...:*
  – This is *the most* interesting neuroradiology case that I *have ever seen.*

- The *first (second, third ...) time ...:*
  – This is the *first time* that I *have seen* a CT of a vertebral hemangiopericytoma

Present Perfect Continuous

Shows an action that began in the past and has gone on up to the present time.

FORM	*Have/has been* + gerund.

USES	<ul><li>To talk about an action that began in the past and has recently stopped or just stopped: – You look tired. *Have you been working* all night? – No, I *have been writing* an article on intussusception reduction using an air enema.</li><li>To ask or say how long something has been happening. In this case the action or situation began in the past and is still happening or has just stopped. – Dr. Sancho and Dr. Martos *have been working* together on the project *from* the beginning.</li></ul>

We use the following particles:

- *How long ...?* (to ask how long):
  - *How long* have you been working as an X-ray technician?

- *For, since* (to say how long):
  - I have been working *for* ten years.
  - I have been working very hard *since* I got this grant.

- *For* (to say how long as a period of time):
  - I have been doing MR imaging *for* three years.

Do not use *for* in expressions with *all*: "I have been working as a radiologist *all* my life" (not "*for all* my life").

- *Since* (to say the beginning of a period):
  - I have been teaching hip ultrasound *since* 1991.

In the present perfect continuous the important thing is the action itself and it does not matter whether the action is finished or not. The action can be finished (just finished) or not (still happening).

In the present perfect the important thing is the result of the action and not the action itself. The action is completely finished.

Past Perfect

Shows an action that happened in the past before another past action. It is the past of the present perfect.

Had + past participle of the verb.

- To say that something had already happened before something else happened:
  - When I arrived at the IR suite, the interventional radiologist *had* already *begun* the aortic aneurysm stenting.

Past Perfect Continuous

Shows an action that began in the past and went on up to a time in the past. It is the past of the present perfect continuous.

FORM	*Had been* + gerund of the verb.

USES	• To say how long something had been happening before something else happened: – She *had been working* as a pediatric radiologist for forty years before she was awarded the Roentgen prize.

Subjunctive

Imagine this situation:

- The surgeon says to the radiologist, "Why don't you do a CT scan on the patient with acute abdominal pain?"
- The surgeon proposes (that) the radiologist do a CT scan on the patient with acute abdominal pain.

The subjunctive is formed always with the base form of the verb (the infinitive without to):

- I suggest (that) you *work* harder.
- She recommended (that) he *give up* smoking while dictating.
- He insisted (that) she *perform an ultrasound examination on* the patient as soon as possible.
- He demanded (that) the nurse *treat him* more politely.

Note that the subjunctive of the verb *to be* is usually passive:

- He insisted (that) the CT *be dictated* immediately.

You can use the subjunctive after:

- Propose
- Suggest
- Recommend
- Insist
- Demand

You can use the subjunctive for the past, present or future:

- He *suggested* (that) the resident *change* the treatment.
- He *recommends* (that) his patients *give up* smoking.

Should is sometimes used instead of the subjunctive:

- The doctor recommended that *I should have* an MRI examination; he suspects that my meniscus is probably torn.

Wish, If Only, Would

Wish

- *Wish* + simple past. To say that we regret something (i.e., that something is not as we would like it to be) in the present:
  - *I wish I were* not on call tomorrow (but I am on call tomorrow).

- *Wish* + past perfect. To say that we regret something that happened or didn't happen in the past:
  - *I wish he hadn't treated* the patient's family so badly (but he treated the patient's family badly).

- *Wish* + *would* + infinitive without *to* when we want something to happen or change or somebody to do something:
  - *I wish you wouldn't dictate* so slowly (note that the speaker is complaining about the present situation or the way people do things).

If Only
If only can be used in exactly the same way as *wish*. It has the same meaning as *wish* but is more dramatic:

- *If only* + past simple (expresses regret in the present):
  - *If only I were not* on call tomorrow.

- *If only* + past perfect (expresses regret in the past):
  - *If only he hadn't treated* the patient's family so badly.

After *wish* and *if only* we use *were* (with I, he, she, it) instead of *was*, and we do not normally use *would*, although sometimes it is possible, or *would have*.

When referring to the present or future, *wish* and *if only* are followed by a past tense, and when referring to the past by a past perfect tense.

Would
Would is used:

- As a modal verb in offers, invitations and requests (i.e., to ask someone to do something):
  - *Would* you help me to write an article on hepatic cholangiocarcinoma? (request).

- *Would* you like to come to the residents' party tonight? (offer and invitation).
- After *wish* (see *Wish*).
- In *if* sentences (see *Conditionals*).
- Sometimes as the past of *will* (in reported speech):
  - Dr. Smith: I will do your bladder ultrasound next week.
  - Patient: The doctor said that he *would* do my bladder ultrasound next week.
- When you remember things that often happened (similar to *used to*):
  - When we were residents, we used to prepare the clinical cases together.
  - When we were residents, we *would* prepare the clinical cases together.

Modal Verbs

FORM

- A modal verb has always the same form.
- There is no -s ending in the third person singular, no -*ing* form and no -*ed* form.
- After a modal verb we use the infinitive without *to* (i.e., the base form of the verb).

These are the English modal verbs:
- *Can* (past form is *could*)
- *Could* (also a modal with its own meaning)
- *May* (past form is *might*)
- *Might* (also a modal with its own meaning)
- *Will*
- *Would*
- *Shall*
- *Should*
- *Ought to*
- *Must*
- *Need*
- *Dare*

We use modal verbs to talk about:
- Ability
- Necessity
- Possibility
- Certainty
- Permission
- Obligation

Expressing Ability

To express ability we can use:

- *Can* (only in the present tense)
- *Could* (only in the past tense)
- *Be able to* (in all tenses)

Ability in the Present

Can (more usual) or *am/is/are able to* (less usual):

- Dr. Williams *can* stent on extremely difficult mesenteric artery stenosis.
- Dr. Rihsnah *is able to* dilate esophagic stenosis in children.
- *Can* you speak medical English? Yes, I *can.*
- *Are you able to* speak medical English? Yes, I am.

Ability in the Past

Could (past form of *can*) or *was/were able to.*

We use *could* to say that someone had the *general* ability to do something:

- When I was a resident I *could* speak German.

We use *was/were able to* to say that someone managed to do something in one particular situation (*specific* ability to do something):

- When I was a resident I *was able to* do fifteen duties in one month.

Managed to can replace *was able to*:

- When I was a resident I *managed to* do fifteen duties in one month.

We use *could have* to say that we had the ability to do something but we didn't do it:

- He *could have* been a surgeon but he became a radiologist instead.

Sometimes we use *could* to talk about ability in a situation which we are imagining (here *could* = *would be able to*):

- I couldn't do your job. I'm not clever enough.

We use *will be able to* to talk about ability with a future meaning:

- If you keep on studying radiological English you *will be able to* write articles for *Radiographics* very soon.

Expressing Necessity

Necessity means that you cannot avoid doing something.

To say that it is necessary to do something we can use *must* or *have to*.

- Necessity in the present: *must, have/has to*.
- Necessity in the past: *had to*.
- Necessity in the future: *must* or *will have to*.

Notice that to express necessity in the past we do not use *must*.

There are some differences between *must* and *have to*:

- We use *must* when the speaker is expressing personal feelings or authority, saying what he or she thinks is necessary:
  - Your chest X-ray film shows severe emphysema. You *must* give up
    smoking.
- We use *have to* when the speaker is not expressing personal feelings or
  authority. The speaker is just giving facts or expressing the authority of
  another person (external authority), often a law or a rule:
  - All radiology residents *have to* learn how to dictate the different types
    of imaging examinations in their first year of residency.

If we want to express that there is necessity to avoid doing something, we
use *mustn't* (i.e., *not allowed to*):

- You *mustn't* eat anything before the intravenous administration of contrast agent.

Expressing No Necessity

To express that there is no necessity we can use the negative forms of *need*
or *have to*:

- No necessity in the present: *needn't* or *don't/doesn't have to*.
- No necessity in the past: *didn't need, didn't have to*.
- No necessity in the future: *won't have to*.

Notice that "there is no necessity to do something" is completely different
from "there is a necessity not to do something".

In conclusion, we use *mustn't* when we are not allowed to do something or
when there is a necessity not to do it, and we use the negative form of
have to or *needn't* when there is no necessity to do something but we can
do it if we want to:

- The radiologist says *I mustn't* get overtired before the procedure but *I needn't* stay in bed.
- The radiologist says *I mustn't* get overtired before the procedure but *I don't have to* stay in bed.

Expressing Possibility

To express possibility we can use *can, could, may* or *might* (from more to less certainty: can, may, might, could).

But also note that "can" is used of ability (or capacity) to do something; "may" of permission or sanction to do it.

Possibility in the Present

To say that something is possible we use *can, may, might, could*:

- High doses of radiation *can* cause you to get cancer (high level of certainty).
- Radiation *may* actually cause you to get cancer (moderate to high level of certainty).
- Radiation *might* cause you to get thyroid cancer (moderate to low level of certainty).
- Radiation *could* cause you to get an osteosarcoma (low level of certainty).

Possibility in the Past

To say that something was possible in the past we use *may have, might have, could have*:

- The lesion *might have* been detected on CT if the slice thickness had been thinner.

Could have is also used to say that something was a possibility or opportunity but it didn't happen:

- You were lucky to be treated with coil embolization, otherwise you *could have* died.

I *couldn't have* done something (i.e., I wouldn't have been able to do it if I had wanted or tried to do it):

- She *couldn't have* seen that mediastinal lesion on the chest X-ray anyway, because it was extremely small.

Possibility in the Future

To talk about possible future actions or happenings we use *may, might, could* (especially in suggestions):

- I don't know where to do my last six months of residency. I *may/might* go to the States.
- We *could* meet later in the hospital to write the article, couldn't we?

When we are talking about possible future plans we can also use the continuous form *may/might/could be + -ing* form:

- I *could be going* to the next RSNA meeting.

Expressing Certainty

To say we are sure that something is true we use *must*:

- You have been reporting all night. You *must* be very tired (i.e., I am sure that you are tired).

To say that we think something is impossible we use *can't*:

- According to his clinical situation and imaging studies, that diagnosis *can't* be true (i.e., I am sure that that diagnosis is not true).

For past situations we use *must have* and *can't have*. We can also use *couldn't have* instead of *can't have*:

- Taking into consideration the situation, the family of the patient *couldn't have* asked for more.

Remember that to express certainty we can also use *will*:

- The double-contrast upper gastrointestinal tract protocol *will* vary from institution to institution.

Expressing Permission

To talk about permission we can use *can, may* (more formal than *can*) or *be allowed to.*

Permission in the Present

Can, may or *am/is/are allowed to:*

- You *can* smoke if you like.
- You *are allowed to* smoke.
- You *may* attend the Congress.

Permission in the Past

Was/were allowed to:

- *Were you allowed to* go into the interventional radiology suite without surgical scrubs?

Permission in the Future

Will be allowed to:

- I *will be allowed to* leave the hospital when my duty is finished.

To ask for permission we use *can, may, could* or *might* (from less to more formal) but not *be allowed to*:

- Hi Hannah, *can* I borrow your digital camera? (if you are asking for a friend's digital camera).
- Dr. Ho, *may* I borrow your digital camera? (if you are talking to an acquaintance).
- *Could* I use your digital camera, Dr. Coltrane? (if you are talking to a colleague you do not know at all).
- *Might* I use your digital camera, Dr. De Roos? (if you are asking for the chairman's digital camera).

Expressing Obligation or Giving Advice

Obligation means that something is the right thing to do.
When we want to say what we think is a good thing to do or the right thing to do we use *should* or *ought to* (a little stronger than *should*).

Should and *ought to* can be used for giving advice:

- You *ought to* sleep.
- You *should* work out.
- You *ought to* give up smoking.
- *Should* he see a doctor? Yes, I think he should.

Conditionals

Conditional sentences have two parts:

1. "If-clause"
2. Main clause

In the sentence "If I were you I would go to the annual meeting of radiology residents", "If I were you" is the if-clause, and "I would go to the annual meeting of radiology residents" is the main clause.

The if-clause can come before or after the main clause. We often put a comma when the if-clause comes first.

Main Types of Conditional Sentences

Type 0

To talk about things that always are true (general truths).

If + simple present + simple present:

- *If* you inject intravenous contrast material, the vessels show high density on a CT scan.
- *If* you see free air in the abdomen, the patient is perforated.
- *If* you drink too much alcohol, you get a sore head.
- *If* you take drugs habitually, you become addicted.

Note that the examples above refer to things that are normally true. They make no reference to the future; they represent a present simple concept. This is the basic (or classic) form of the conditional type 0.

There are possible variations of this form. In the if-clause and in the main clause we can use the present continuous, present perfect simple or present perfect continuous instead of the present simple. In the main clause we can also use the imperative instead of the present simple:

- Residents only get a certificate *if* they *have attended* the course regularly.

So the type 0 form can be reduced to:

- *If* + present form + present form or imperative.

Present forms include the present simple, present continuous, present perfect simple, and present perfect continuous.

Type 1

To talk about future situations that the speaker thinks are likely to happen (the speaker is thinking about a real possibility in the future).

If + simple present + future simple (*will*):

- *If* I find something new about the percutaneous treatment of malignant obstructive jaundice, I will tell you.

- *If* we analyze contrast agents, we will be able to infer laws and principles about their effect over renal function.

These examples refer to future things that are possible and it is quite probable that they will happen. This is the basic (or classic) form of the conditional type 1.

There are possible variations of the basic form. In the if-clause we can use the present continuous, the present perfect or the present perfect continuous instead of the present simple. In the main clause we can use the future continuous, future perfect simple or future perfect continuous instead of the future simple. Modals such as *can*, *may* or *might* are also possible.

So the form of type 1 can be reduced to:

- *If* + present form + future form

Future forms include the future simple, future continuous, future perfect simple, and future perfect continuous.

Type 2

To talk about future situations that the speaker thinks are possible but not probable (the speaker is imagining a possible future situation) or to talk about unreal situations in the present.

If + simple past + conditional (*would*):

- Peter, *if* you *studied* harder, you *would* be better prepared for doing your CAQ in neuroradiology.

The above sentence tells us that Peter is supposed not to be studying hard.

- *If* I *were* you, I *would* go to the Annual Meeting of Interventional Radiology (but I am not you).
- *If* I *were* a resident again I *would* go to Harvard Medical School for a whole year to complete my training period (but I am not a resident).

There are possible variations of the basic form. In the if-clause we can use the past continuous instead of the past simple. In the main clause we can use *could* or *might* instead of *would*.

So the form of type 2 can be reduced to:

- *If* + past simple or continuous + *would*, *could* or *might*.

Type 3

To talk about past situations that didn't happen (impossible actions in the past).

If + past perfect + perfect conditional (*would have*):

- *If* I *had known* the patient's symptoms, *I would* probably *have* not missed the small pancreatic lesion on the CT scan.

As you can see, we are talking about the past. The real situation is that I didn't know the patient's symptoms so that I didn't notice the small pancreatic lesion.

This is the basic (or classic) form of the third type of conditional. There are possible variations. In the if-clause we can use the past perfect continuous instead of the past perfect simple. In the main clause we can use the continuous form of the perfect conditional instead of the perfect conditional simple. *Would probably, could* or *might* instead of *would* are also possible (when we are not sure about something).

In Case

"The interventional radiologist wears two pairs of latex gloves during an intervention *in case* one of them tears." *In case one of them tears* because it is possible that one of them tears during the intervention (in the future).

Note that we don't use *will* after *in case*. We use a present tense after *in case* when we are talking about the future.

In case is not the same as *if*. Compare these sentences:

- We'll buy some more food and drink *if* the new residents come to our department's party. (Perhaps the new residents will come to our party. If they come, we will buy some more food and drink; if they don't come, we won't.)
- We will buy some food and drink *in case* the new residents come to our department's party. (Perhaps the new residents will come to our department's party. We will buy some more food and drink whether they come or not.)

We can also use *in case* to say why someone did something in the past:

- He rang the bell again *in case* the nurse hadn't heard it the first time. (Because it was possible that the nurse hadn't heard it the first time.)
  In case of (= if there is):
- *In case of* pregnancy, don't have an X-ray examination.

Unless

"Don't take these pills *unless* you are extremely anxious." (Don't take these pills except if you are extremely anxious.) This sentence means that you can take the pills only if you are extremely anxious.

We use *unless* to make an exception to something we say. In the example above the exception is *you are extremely anxious*.

We often use *unless* in warnings:

- *Unless* you send the application form today, you won't be accepted in the next National Congress of Radiology.

It is also possible to use *if* in a negative sentence instead of *unless*:

- Don't take those pills *if you aren't* extremely anxious.
- *If you don't send* the application form today, you won't be accepted in the next Congress of Radiology.

As Long As, Provided (That), Providing (That)

These expressions mean *but only if*:

- You can use my new pen to sign your report *as long as* you write carefully (i.e., *but only if* you write carefully).
- Going by car to the hospital is convenient *provided* (*that*) you have somewhere to park (i.e., *but only if* you have somewhere to park).
- *Providing* (*that*) she studies the clinical cases, she will deliver a bright presentation.

Passive Voice

Study these examples:

- The first ultrasound examination was performed at our hospital in 1980 (passive sentence).
- Someone performed the first ultrasound examination at our hospital in 1980 (active sentence).

Both sentences are correct and mean the same. They are two different ways of saying the same thing, but in the passive sentence we try to make the object of the active sentence ("the first ultrasound examination") more important by putting it at the beginning. So, we prefer to use the passive when it is not that important who or what did the action. In the example above, it is not so important (or not known) who performed the first ultrasound examination.

Active sentence:

- Fleming (subject) discovered (active verb) penicillin (object) in 1950.
  Passive sentence:

- Penicillin (subject) was discovered (passive verb) by Fleming (agent) in 1950.

The passive verb is formed by putting the verb *to be* into the same tense as the active verb and adding the past participle of the active verb:

- Discovered (active verb) – was discovered (*be* + past participle of the active verb).

The object of an active verb becomes the subject of the passive verb ("penicillin"). The subject of an active verb becomes the agent of the passive verb ("Fleming"). We can leave out the agent if it is not important to mention it or we don't know it. If we want to mention it, we will put it at the end of the sentence preceded by the particle *by* ("... by Fleming").

Some sentences have two objects, indirect and direct. In these sentences the passive subject can be either the direct object or the indirect object of the active sentence:

- The doctor gave the patient a new treatment.

There are two possibilities:

- A new treatment was given to the patient.
- The patient was given a new treatment.

Passive Forms of Present and Past Tenses

Simple Present

Active:
- Radiologists review the most interesting cases in the clinical session every day.

Passive:
- The most interesting cases are reviewed in the clinical session every day.

Simple Past

Active:
- The nurse checked the renal function of the patient before the CT examination.

Passive:
- The renal function of the patient was checked before the CT examination.

Present Continuous

Active:
- Dr. Golightly is reporting an intravenous urogram right now.

Passive:
- An intravenous urogram is being reported right now.

Past Continuous

Active:
- They were carrying the injured person to the CT room.

Passive:
- The injured person was being carried to the CT room.

Present Perfect

Active:
- The radiologist has performed ten lower-extremity Doppler ultrasounds this morning.

Passive:
- Ten lower-extremity Doppler ultrasounds have been performed this morning.

Past Perfect

Active:
- They had sent the CT films before the operation started.

Passive:
- The CT films had been sent before the operation started.

In sentences of the type "people say/consider/know/think/believe/expect/ understand ... that ...", such as "Doctors consider that AIDS is a fatal disease", we have two possible passive forms:

- AIDS is considered to be a fatal disease.
- It is considered that AIDS is a fatal disease.

Have/Get Something Done

FORM	*Have/get* + object + past participle.

Get is a little more informal than *have*, and it is often used in informal spoken English:

- You should *get* your ultrasound machine tested.
- You should *have* your ultrasound machine tested.

When we want to say that we don't want to do something ourselves and we arrange for someone to do it for us, we use the expression *have something done*:

- The patient had all his metal objects removed in order to prevent accidents during the MR examination.

Sometimes the expression *have something done* has a different meaning:

- John had his knee broken playing a football match. MRI showed a meniscal tear.

It is obvious that this doesn't mean that he arranged for somebody to break his knee. With this meaning, we use *have something done* to say that something (often something not nice) happened to someone.

Supposed To

Supposed to can be used in the following ways:

Can be used like *said to*:
- The chairman is supposed to be the one who runs the department.

To say what is planned or arranged (and this is often different from what really happens):

- The fourth year resident is supposed to read this CT.

To say what is not allowed or not advisable:
- She was not supposed to be on call yesterday.

Reported Speech

Imagine that you want to tell someone else what the patient said. You can either repeat the patient's words or use reported speech.

The reporting verb (*said* in the examples below) can come before or after the reported clause (*there was a conference about cardiac MR that evening*), but it usually comes before the reported clause. When the reporting verb comes before, we can use *that* to introduce the reported clause or we can leave it out (leaving it out is more informal). When the reporting verb comes after, we cannot use *that* to introduce the reported clause.

The reporting verb can report statements and thoughts, questions, orders, and requests.

Reporting in the Present

When the reporting verb is in the present tense, it isn't necessary to change the tense of the verb:

- "I'll help you guys with this esophagogram", he says.
- He says (that) he will help us obtain this esophagogram.
- "The vertebroplasty will take place this morning", he says.
- He says (that) the vertebroplasty will take place this morning.

Reporting in the Past

When the reporting verb is in the past tense, the verb in direct speech usually changes in the following ways:

- Simple present changes to simple past.
- Present continuous changes to past continuous.
- Simple past changes to past perfect.
- Past continuous changes to past perfect continuous.
- Present perfect changes to past perfect.
- Present perfect continuous changes to past perfect continuous.
- Past perfect stays the same.
- Future changes to conditional.
- Future continuous changes to conditional continuous.
- Future perfect changes to conditional perfect.
- Conditional stays the same.
- Present forms of modal verbs stay the same.
- Past forms of modal verbs stay the same.

Pronouns, adjectives and adverbs also change. Here are some examples:

- First person singular changes to third person singular.
- Second person singular changes to first person singular.
- First person plural changes to third person plural.
- Second person plural changes to first person plural.
- Third person singular changes to third person plural.
- Now changes to then.
- Today changes to that day.
- Tomorrow changes to the day after.
- Yesterday changes to the day before.
- This changes to that.
- Here changes to there.
- Ago changes to before.

It is not always necessary to change the verb when you use reported speech. If you are reporting something and you feel that it is still true, you do not need to change the tense of the verb, but if you want you can do it:

- The treatment of choice for severe urticaria after intravenous contrast administration is epinephrine.
- He said (that) the treatment of choice for severe urticaria after intravenous contrast administration is epinephrine.

or

- He said (that) the treatment of choice for severe urticaria after intravenous contrast administration was epinephrine.

Reporting Questions

Yes and No Questions

We use *whether* or *if*:

- Do you smoke or drink any alcohol?
- The doctor asked if I smoked or drank any alcohol.

- Have you had any urticaria after intravenous contrast injections?
- The doctor asked me whether I had had any urticaria after intravenous contrast injections or not.

- Are you taking any pills or medicines at the moment?
- The doctor asked me if I was taking any pills or medicines at that moment.

Wh ... Questions

We use the same question word as in the *wh* ... question:

- What do you mean by saying you are feeling under the weather?
- The doctor asked me what I meant by saying I was feeling under the weather.

- Why do you think you feel under the weather?
- The doctor asked me why I thought I felt under the weather.

- When do you feel under the weather?
- The doctor asked me when I felt under the weather.

- How often do you have headaches?
- The doctor asked how often I had headaches.

Reported Questions

Reported questions have the following characteristics:

- The word order is different from that of the original question. The verb follows the subject as in an ordinary statement.

- The auxiliary verb *do* is not used.
- There is no question mark.
- The verb changes in the same way as in direct speech.

Study the following examples:
- How old are you?
- The doctor asked me how old I was.

- Do you smoke?
- The doctor asked me if I smoked.

Reporting Orders and Requests

<table>
<tr><td>FORM</td><td>*Tell* (pronoun) + object (indirect) + infinitive:
• Take the pills before meals.
• The doctor told me to take the pills before meals.
• You mustn't smoke.
• The doctor told me not to smoke.</td></tr>
</table>

Reporting Suggestions and Advice

Suggestions and advice are reported in the following forms:

- Suggestions
  - Why don't we operate on that patient this evening?
  - The surgeon suggested operating on that patient that evening.

- Advice
  - You had better stay in bed.
  - The doctor advised me to stay in bed.

Questions

In sentences with *to be*, *to have* (in its auxiliary form) and modal verbs, we usually make questions by changing the word order:

- Affirmative
  - You are a radiologist.
  - Interrogative: Are you a radiologist?

- Negative
  - You are not a radiologist.
  - Interrogative: Aren't you a radiologist?

In simple present questions we use *do/does*:

- His stomach hurts after having barium for upper GI examination.
- Does his stomach hurt after having barium for upper GI examination?

In simple past questions we use *did*:

- The nurse arrived on time.
- Did the nurse arrive on time?

If *who/what/which* is the subject of the sentence we do not use *do*:

- Someone paged Dr. W.
- Who paged Dr. W?

If *who/what/which* is the object of the sentence we use *did*:

- Dr. W. paged someone.
- Who did Dr. W. page?

When we ask somebody and begin the question with *Do you know ...* or *Could you tell me ...* , the rest of the question maintains the affirmative sentence's word order:

- Where is the reading room?

but

- Do you know where the reading room is?

- Where is the library?

but

- Could you tell me where the library is?

Reported questions also maintain the affirmative sentence's word order:

- Dr. Wilson asked: How are you?

but

- Dr. Wilson asked me how I was.

Short answers are possible in questions where *be, do, can, have* and *might* are auxiliary verbs:

- Do you smoke? Yes, I do.
- Did you smoke? No, I didn't.
- Can you walk? Yes, I can.

We also use auxiliary verbs with *so* (affirmative) and *neither* or *nor* (negative) changing the word order:

- I am feeling tired. So am I.
- I can't remember the name of the disease. Neither can I.
- Is he going to pass the boards? I think so.

- Will you be on call tomorrow? I guess not.
- Will you be off call the day after tomorrow? I hope so.
- Has the Chairman been invited to the party? I'm afraid so.

Tag questions

We use a positive tag question with a negative sentence and vice versa:

- The first year resident isn't feeling very well today, is she?
- You are working late at the lab, aren't you?

After *let's* the tag question is *shall we*?

- Let's read a couple of articles, shall we?

After the imperative, the tag question is *will you*?

- Turn off the viewer, will you?

Infinitive/-Ing

Verb + -Ing

There are certain verbs that are usually used in the structure verb + -*ing* when followed by another verb:

- *Stop*: Please *stop talking*.
- *Finish*: *I've finished translating* the article into English.
- *Enjoy*: I *enjoy talking* to patients while I'm doing an ultrasound on them.
- *Mind*: I *don't mind being* told what to do.
- *Suggest*: Dr. Knight *suggested going* to the OT and trying to operate on the aneurysm that we couldn't stent.
- *Dislike*: She *dislikes going* out late after a night on-call.
- *Imagine*: I *can't imagine you operating*. You told me you hate blood.
- *Regret*: He *regrets having gone* two minutes before his patient had seizures.
- *Admit*: The resident *admitted forgetting* to report Mrs. Smith's mammography.
- *Consider*: Have you *considered finishing* your residence in the USA?

Other verbs that follow this structure are: *avoid, deny, involve, practice, miss, postpone,* and *risk*.

The following expressions also take -*ing*:

- *Give up*: Are you going to *give up smoking*?

- *Keep on*: She *kept on interrupting* me while I was speaking.
- *Go on*: *Go on studying*, the exam will be next month.

When we are talking about finished actions, we can also use the verb *to have*:

- The resident *admitted forgetting* to report Mrs. Smith's mammography.

or

- The resident *admitted having forgotten* to report Mrs. Smith's mammography.

And, with some of these verbs (*admit*, *deny*, *regret* and *suggest*), you also can use a "that ..." structure:

- The resident *admitted forgetting* to report Mrs. Smith's mammography.

or

- The resident *admitted that he had forgotten* to report Mrs. Smith's mammography.

Verb + Infinitive

When followed by another verb, these verbs are used with verb + infinitive structure:

- *Agree*: The patient *agreed to give up* smoking.
- *Refuse*: The patient *refused to give up* smoking.
- *Promise*: I *promised to give up* smoking.
- *Threaten*: Dr. Sommerset *threatened to close* the radiology department.
- *Offer*: The unions *offered to negotiate*.
- *Decide*: Dr. Knight's patients *decided to leave* the waiting room.

Other verbs that follow this structure are: *attempt, manage, fail, plan, arrange, afford, forget, learn, dare, tend, appear, seem, pretend, need,* and *intend*.

There are two possible structures after these verbs: *want, ask, expect, help, would like,* and *would prefer*:

- Verb + infinitive: I *asked to see* Dr. Knight, the surgeon who operated on my patient.
- Verb + object + infinitive: I *asked Dr. Knight to inform* me about my patient.

There is only one possible structure after the following verbs: *tell, order, remind, warn, force, invite, enable, teach, persuade,* and *get*:

- Verb + object + infinitive: *Remind me to report* those radiographs tomorrow before 10 a.m.

There are two possible structures after the following verbs:

- *Advise*:
    - I *wouldn't advise learning* at that radiology department.
    - I *wouldn't advise you to learn* at that radiology department.

- *Allow*:
    - They *don't allow smoking* in the CT room.
    - They *don't allow you to smoke* in the CT room.

- *Permit*:
    - They *don't permit eating* in the radiology reading room.
    - They *don't permit you to eat* in the radiology reading room.

When you use *make* and *let*, you should use the structure: verb + base form (instead of verb + infinitive):

- Blood *makes me feel* dizzy (you can't say: blood *makes me to feel* ...).
- Dr. Knight *wouldn't let me stent on* his patient.

After the following expressions and verbs you can use either *-ing* or the infinitive: *like, hate, love, can't stand,* and *can't bear*:

- She *can't stand being* alone while she is performing an ultrasound examination.
- She *can't stand to be* alone while she is performing an ultrasound examination.

After the following verbs you can use *-ing* but not the infinitive: *dislike, enjoy,* and *mind*:

- I *enjoy being* alone (not: I *enjoy to be alone*).
    Would like, a polite way of saying *I want,* is followed by the infinitive:
- *Would you like to be* the chairman of the neuroimaging division?

Begin, start and *continue* can be followed by either *-ing* or the infinitive:

- The patient *began to improve* after the percutaneous drainage of his collection.
- The patient *began improving* after the percutaneous drainage of his collection.

With some verbs, such as *remember* and *try*, the use of *-ing* and infinitive after them have different meanings:

- *Remember*:
    - *I did not remember to place* the tip of the catheter at the IVC before starting the contrast injection (I forgot to place the catheter properly).
    - *I could remember (myself) placing* the tip of a catheter at the IVC that day (I can recall placing the catheter).

- *Try*:
  - The patient *tried to keep* her eyes open while the MR examination was going on.
  - If your headache persists, *try asking for* a MRI.

Verb + Preposition + -*Ing*

If a verb comes after a preposition, that verb ends in -*ing*:

- Are you *interested in working* for our hospital?
- *What are the advantages of developing* new radiological techniques?
- *She's not very good at learning* languages.

You can use -*ing* with *before* and *after*:

- Discharge Mr. Brown *before operating* on the aneurysm.
- What did you do *after finishing* your residence?

You can use *by* + -*ing* to explain how something happened:

- You can improve your medical English *by reading* scientific articles.

You can use -*ing* after *without*:

- Jim got to the hospital *without realizing* he had left his locker keys at home.

Be careful with *to* because it can either be a part of the infinitive or a preposition:

- I'm looking forward to see you again (this is NOT correct).
- I'm looking forward to seeing you again.
- I'm looking forward to the next European congress.

Review the following verb + preposition expressions:

- *succeed in* finding a job
- *feel like* going out tonight
- *think about* operating on that patient
- *dream of* being a radiologist
- *disapprove of* smoking
- *look forward to* hearing from you
- *insist on* inviting me to chair the session
- *apologize for* keeping Dr. Ho waiting
- *accuse* (someone) *of* telling lies
- *suspected of* having AIDS
- *stop from* leaving the ward
- *thank* (someone) *for* being helpful
- *forgive* (someone) *for* not writing to me
- *warn* (someone) *against* carrying on smoking

The following are some examples of expressions + *-ing*:

- *I don't feel like* going out tonight.
- *It's no use* trying to persuade her.
- *There's no point in* waiting for him.
- *It's not worth* taking a taxi. The hospital is only a short walk from here.
- *It's worth* looking again at that radiograph.
- *I am having difficulty* reporting that T-tube cholangiogram
- *I am having trouble* reporting that T-tube cholangiogram.

Countable and Uncountable Nouns

Countable Nouns

Countable nouns are things we can count. We can make them plural.

Before singular countable nouns you may use *a/an*:
- You will be attended to by *a* radiologist.
- Dr. Vida is looking for *an* anesthetist.

Remember to use *a/an* for jobs:
- I'm *a* radiologist.

Before plural countable nouns you use *some* as a general rule:

- I've read *some* good articles on spiral chest CT lately.

    Don't use *some* when you are talking about general things:
- Generally speaking, I like radiology books.

You have to use *some* when you mean some, but not all:

- *Some* doctors carry a stethoscope but radiologists don't.

Uncountable Nouns

Uncountable nouns are things we cannot count. They have no plural.

You cannot use *a/an* before an uncountable noun; in this case you have to use *the, some, any, much, this, his,* etc ... or leave the uncountable noun alone, without the article:

- The chairman gave me an advice (NOT correct).
- The chairman gave me *some* advice.

Many nouns can be used as countable or uncountable nouns. Usually there is a difference in their meaning:

- I had *many experiences* on my rotation at the Children's Hospital (countable).
- I need *experience* to become a good radiologist (uncountable).

Some nouns are uncountable in English but often countable in other languages: *advice, baggage, behavior, bread, chaos, furniture, information, luggage, news, permission, progress, scenery, traffic, travel, trouble,* and *weather.*

Articles: *A/An* and *The*

The speaker says *a/an* when it is the first time he talks about something, but once the listener knows what the speaker is talking about, he says *the*:

- This morning I did *an* ultrasound and *a* chest plain film. *The* ultrasound was completely normal.

We use *the* when it is clear which thing or person we mean:

- Can you turn off *the* light.
- Where is *the* radiology chest division, please?

As a general rule, we say:

- The police
- The bank
- The post office
- The fire department
- The doctor
- The hospital
- The dentist

We say: *the* sea, *the* sky, *the* ground, *the* city, and *the* country.

We don't use *the* with the names of meals:

- What did you have for lunch/breakfast/dinner?

But we use *a* when there is an adjective before a noun:

- Thank you. It was *a* delicious dinner.

We use *the* for musical instruments:

- Can you play *the* piano?

We use *the* with absolute adjectives (adjectives used as nouns). The meaning is always plural. For example:

- The rich
- The old
- The blind
- The sick
- The disabled
- The injured
- The poor
- The young
- The deaf
- The dead
- The unemployed
- The homeless

We use *the* with nationality words (note that nationality words always begin with a capital letter):

- *The* British, *the* Dutch, *the* Spanish.

We don't use *the* before a noun when we mean something in general:

- I love doctors (not the doctors).

With the words *school, college, prison, jail, church* we use *the* when we mean the buildings and leave the substantives alone otherwise. We say: *go to bed, go to work* and *go home*. We don't use *the* in these cases.

We use *the* with geographical names according to the following rules:

- Continents don't use *the*:
  - Our new resident comes from Asia.
- Countries/states don't use *the*:
  - The patient that underwent a liver duplex ultrasound came from Sweden.
  (except for country names that include words such as Republic, Kingdom, States ... ; e.g., the United States of America, the United Kingdom, and The Netherlands).

As a general rule, cities don't use *the*:

- The next Radiology Congress will be held in Zaragoza.

Islands don't use *the* with individual islands but do use it with groups:

- Dr. Holmes comes from Sicily and her husband from the Canary Islands.

Lakes don't use *the*; oceans, seas, rivers and canals do use it.

- Lake Windermere is beautiful.
- *The* Panama canal links *the* Atlantic ocean to *the* Pacific ocean.

We use *the* with streets, buildings, airports, universities, etc, according to the following rules:

- Streets, roads, avenues, boulevards and squares don't use *the*:
  – The hospital is sited at 15th. Avenue.
- Airports don't use *the*:
  – The plane arrived at JFK airport
- We use *the* before publicly recognized buildings: *the* White House, *the* Empire State Building, *the* Louvre museum, *the* Prado museum.
- We use *the* before names with of: *the* Tower of London, *the* Great Wall of China.
- Universities don't use *the*: I studied at Harvard.

Word Order

The order of adjectives is discussed in the section Adjectives under the heading Adjective Order

The *verb* and the *object* of the verb normally go together:

- I studied radiology because I like *watching images* very much (*not* I like very much watching images).

We usually say the place before the time:

- She has been practicing interventional radiology in London since April.

We put some adverbs in the middle of the sentence:
If the verb is one word we put the adverb before the verb:

- I performed his carotid duplex ultrasound and *also spoke* to his family.

We put the adverb after *to be*:

- You are *always* on time.

We put the adverb after the first part of a compound verb:

- Are you *definitely* attending the musculoskeletal radiology course?

In negative sentences we put *probably* before the negative:

- I *probably* won't see you at the congress.

We also use *all* and *both* in these positions:

- Jack and Tom are *both* able to carry out a carotid angiogram.
- We *all* felt sick after the meal.

Relative Clauses

A clause is a part of a sentence. A relative clause tells us which person or thing (or what kind of person or thing) the speaker means.

A relative clause (e.g. *who is on call?*) begins with a relative pronoun (e.g. *who, that, which, whose*).

A relative clause comes after a noun phrase (e.g. the doctor, the nurse).

Most relative clauses are defining clauses and some of them are non-defining clauses.

Defining Clauses

- *The book on interventional radiology (that) you lent me is very interesting.*

The relative clause is essential to the meaning of the sentence.

Commas are not used to separate the relative clause from the rest of the sentence.

That is often used instead of *who* or *which*, especially in speech.

If the relative pronoun is the object (direct object) of the clause, it can be omitted.

If the relative pronoun is the subject of the clause, it cannot be omitted.

Non-Defining Clauses

- *The first vertebral angiogram in Australia, which took place at our hospital, was a complete success.*

The relative clause is not essential to the meaning of the sentence; it gives us additional information.

Commas are usually used to separate the relative clause from the rest of the sentence.

That cannot be used instead of *who* or *which*.

The relative pronoun cannot be omitted.

Relative Pronouns

Relative pronouns are used for people and for things.

- For people:
    - Subject: *who, that*
    - Object: *who, that, whom*
    - Possessive: *whose*

- For things:
  - Subject: *which, that*
  - Object: *which, that*
  - Possessive: *whose*

Who is used only for people. It can be the subject or the object of a relative clause:

- The patient *who* was admitted in a shock situation is getting better. Can we perform the cranial MRI now?

Which is used only for things. Like *who*, it can be the subject or object of a relative clause:

- The materials *which* are used for embolization are very expensive.

That is often used instead of *who* or *which*, especially in speech.

Whom is used only for people. It is grammatically correct as the object of a relative clause, but it is very formal and is not often used in spoken English. We can use *whom* instead of *who* when *who* is the object of the relative clause or when there is a preposition after the verb of the relative clause:

- The resident *who* I am going to the congress with is very nice.
- The resident with *whom* I am going to the congress is a very nice and intelligent person.
- The patient *who* I saw in the Interventional Radiology Department yesterday has been diagnosed with Leriche's syndrome.
- The patient *whom* I saw in the Interventional Radiology Department yesterday has been diagnosed with Leriche's syndrome.

Whose is the possessive relative pronoun. It can be used for people and things. We cannot omit *whose*:

- Nurses *whose* wages are low should be paid more.

We can leave out *who, which* or *that*:

- When it is the object of a relative clause.
  - The article on the spleen that you wrote is great.
  - The article on splenic embolization you wrote is great.
- When there is a preposition. Remember that, in a relative clause, we usually put a preposition in the same place as in the main clause (after the verb):
  - The congress that we are going to next week is very expensive.
  - The congress we are going to next week is very expensive.

Prepositions in Relative Clauses

We can use a preposition in a relative clause with *who, which,* or *that,* or without a pronoun.

In relative clauses we put a preposition in the same place as in a main clause (after the verb). We don't usually put it before the relative pronoun. This is the normal order in informal spoken English:

- This is a problem *which* we can do very little about.
- The nurse (*who*) I spoke to earlier isn't here now.

In more formal or written English we can put a preposition at the beginning of a relative clause. But if we put a preposition at the beginning, we can only use *which* or *whom.* We cannot use the pronouns *that* or *who* after a preposition:

- This is a problem *about which* we can do very little.
- The nurse *to whom* I spoke earlier isn't here now.

Relative Clauses Without a Pronoun (Special Cases)

Infinitive Introducing a Clause

We can use the infinitive instead of a relative pronoun and a verb after:

- The first, the second ... and the next
- The only
- Superlatives

For example:
- Roentgen was the first man *to use* X-rays.
- Joe was the only one *to discover* the diagnosis.

-Ing and -Ed Forms Introducing a Clause

We can use an *-ing* form instead of a relative pronoun and an active verb:

- Residents *wanting* to train abroad should have a good level of English.

We can use an *-ed* form instead of a relative pronoun and a passive verb:

- The man *injured* in the accident was taken to the CT room.

The *-ing* form or the *-ed* form can replace a verb in a present or past tense.

Why, When and Where

We can use *why*, *when* and *where* in a defining relative clause.
    We can leave out *why* or *when*. We can also leave out *where*, but then we must use a preposition.

We can form non-defining relative clauses with *when* and *where*:

● The clinical history, *where* everything about a patient is written, is a very important document.
    We cannot leave out *when* and *where* from a non-defining clause.

Adjectives

An adjective describes (tells us something about) a noun.
    In English, adjectives come before nouns (old hospital) and have the same form in both the singular and the plural (new hospital, new hospitals) and in the masculine and in the feminine.

An adjective can be used with certain verbs such as *be, get, seem, appear, look* (meaning *seem*), *feel, sound, taste* ... :

● He has been *ill* since Friday, so he couldn't report that bone age.
● The patient was getting *worse*.
● The ultrasound-guided core biopsy seemed *easy*, but it wasn't.
● The colonic luminogram appears *black* when it is normal.
● You look rather *tired*. Have you tested your RBC?
● She felt *sick*, so she stopped the renal transplant scan.
● Food in hospitals tastes *horrible*.

As you can see, in these examples there is no noun after the adjective.

Adjective Order

We have *fact adjectives* and *opinion adjectives*. Fact adjectives (*large, new, white, ...*) give us objective information about something (size, age, color, ...). Opinion adjectives (*nice, beautiful, intelligent, ...*) tell us what someone thinks of something.

In a sentence, opinion adjectives usually go before fact adjectives:

● An *intelligent* (opinion) *young* (fact) radiologist visited me this morning.
● Dr. Spencer has a *nice* (opinion) *red* (fact) Porsche.

Sometimes there are two or more fact adjectives describing a noun, and generally we put them in the following order:

1. Size/length
2. Shape/width
3. Age
4. Color
5. Nationality
6. Material

For example:

- A tall young nurse
- A small round lesion
- A black latex leaded pair of gloves
- A large new white latex leaded pair of gloves
- An old American patient
- A tall young Italian resident
- A small square old blue iron monitor

Regular Comparison of Adjectives

The form used for a comparison depends upon the number of syllables in the adjective.

Adjectives of One Syllable
One-syllable adjectives (for example *fat, thin, tall*) are used with expressions of the form:

- *less ... than* (inferiority)
- *as ... as* (equality)
- *-er ... than* (superiority)

For example:
- Calls are *less hard than* a few years ago.
- Eating in the hospital is *as cheap as* eating at the Medical School.
- Ultrasound examinations are difficult nowadays because people tend to be *fatter than* in the past.

Adjectives of Two Syllables
Two-syllable adjectives (for example *easy, dirty, clever*) are used with expressions of the form:

- *less ... than* (inferiority)
- *as ... as* (equality)
- *-er/more ... than* (superiority)

We prefer -*er* for adjectives ending in *y* (*easy, funny, pretty* ...) and other adjectives (such as *quiet, simple, narrow, clever* ...). For other two-syllable adjectives we use *more*.

For example:

- The radiological problem is *less simple than* you think.
- My arm is *as painful as* it was yesterday.
- The board exam was *easier than* we expected.
- His illness was *more serious than* we first suspected, as demonstrated on the high-resolution chest CT.

Adjectives of Three or More Syllables

Adjectives of three or more syllables (for example *difficult, expensive, comfortable*) are used with expressions of the form:

- *less ... than* (inferiority)
- *as ... as* (equality)
- *more ... than* (superiority)

For example:

- Studying medicine in Spain is *less expensive than* in the States.
- The small hospital was *as comfortable* as a hotel.
- Studying the case was *more interesting than* I had thought.

Before the comparative of adjectives you can use:

- *a (little) bit*
- *a little*
- *much*
- *a lot*
- *far*

For example:

- I am going to try something *much simpler* to solve the problem.
- The patient is *a little better* today.
- The little boy is *a bit worse* today.

Sometimes it is possible to use two comparatives together (when we want to say that something is changing continuously):

- It is becoming *more and more* difficult to find a job in an academic hospital.

We also say *twice as ... as, three times as ... as*:

- Going to the European Congress of Radiology *is twice as expensive as* going to the French one.

The Superlative

The form used for a superlative depends upon the number of syllables in the adjective:

Adjectives of One Syllable
One-syllable adjectives are used with expressions of the form:

- *the ...-est*
- *the least*

For example:

- The number of radiologists in your country is the *highest* in the world.

Adjectives of Two Syllables
Two-syllable adjectives are used with expressions of the form:

- *the ...-est/the most*
- *the least*

For example:

- Barium enema is one of the *commonest* tests in clinical practice.
- Barium enema is one of the *most common* tests in clinical practice.

Adjectives of Three or More Syllables
Adjectives of three or more syllables are used with:

- *the most*
- *the least*

For example:

- Common sense and patience are *the most important* things for a radiologist.
- This is the *least difficult* brain CT I have reported in years.

Irregular Forms of Adjectives

- good   better the best
- bad   worse the worst
- far farther/further the farthest/furthest

For example:

- My ultrasound technique is *worse* now than during my first year of residence in spite of having attended several ultrasound refresher courses.

Comparatives with *The*

We use *the* + comparative to talk about a change in one thing which causes a change in something else:

- The nearer the X-ray focus the better image we have.
- The more you practice ultrasound the easier it gets.
- The higher the contrast amount the greater the risk of renal failure.

As

Two things happening at the same time or over the same period of time:

- The resident listened carefully *as* Dr. Fraser explained to the patient the different diagnostic possibilities.
- I began to enjoy the residency more *as* I got used to being on call.

One thing happening during another:

- The patient died *as* the CT scan was being performed.
- I had to leave just *as* the differential diagnosis discussion was getting interesting.

Note that we use *as* only if two actions happen together. If one action follows another we don't use *as*, we use the particle *when*:

- *When* the injured person came to the MRI room, I decided to call the surgeon.

Meaning *because*:

- *As* I was feeling sick, I decided to go to the doctor.

Like and *As*

Like

Like is a preposition, so it can be followed by a noun, pronoun or *-ing* form.

It means *similar to* or *the same as*. We use it when we compare things:

- This comfortable head coil is *like* a velvet hat.
- What does he do? He is a radiologist, *like* me.

As

As + subject + verb:

- Don't change the dose of contrast agent. Leave everything *as* it is.
- He should have been treated *as* I showed you.

Meaning *what*:

- The resident did *as* he was told.
- He made the diagnosis just with the chest X-ray, *as* I expected.
- *As* you know, we are sending an article to the European Journal of Radiology next week.
- *As* I thought, the patient was under the influence of alcohol.

As can also be a preposition, so it can be used with a noun, but it has a different meaning from *like*.

As + noun is used to say what something really is or was (especially when we talk about someone's job or how we use something):

- Before becoming a radiologist I worked *as* a general practitioner in a small village.

As if, *as though* are used to say how someone or something looks, sounds, feels, ..., or to say how someone does something:

- The doctor treated me *as if* I were his son.
- John sounds *as though* he has got a cold.

Expressions with *as*:
- *Such as*
- *As usual* (Dr. Mas was late *as usual*.)

So and Such

So and *such* make the meaning of the adjective stronger.

We use *so* with an adjective without a noun or with an adverb:

- The first-year resident is *so clever*.
- The neuroradiologist injected lidocaine *so carefully* that the patient did not notice it.

We use *such* with an adjective with a noun:

- She is *such a clever resident*.

Prepositions

At/On/In Time

We use *at* with times:

- *At* 7 o'clock
- *At* midnight
- *At* breakfast time

We usually leave out *at* when we ask (*at*) *what time*:

- *What time* are you reporting this evening?

We also use *at* in these expressions:

- *At* night
- *At* the moment
- *At* the same time
- *At* the beginning of
- *At* the end of

For example:

- I don't like to be on call *at night*.
- Dr. Knight is reporting some studies *at the moment*.

We use *in* for longer periods of time:

- *In* June
- *In* summer
- *In* 1977

We also say *in the morning, in the afternoon, in the evening*:

- I'll report all the MRI studies *in the morning*.

We use *on* with days and dates:

- *On* October 9th
- *On* Monday
- *On* Saturday mornings
- *On* the weekend (*At* the weekend in British English)

We do not use *at/in/on* before *last* and *next*:

- I'll be on call *next* Saturday.
- They bought a new scanner *last* year.
  We use *in* before a period of time (i.e., a time in the future):

- Our resident went to Boston to do a rotation on abdominal imaging. He'll be back *in* a year.

For, During **and** While

We use *for* to say to how long something takes:

- I've worked as a radiologist at this hospital *for* ten years.

You cannot use *during* in this way:

- It rained *for* five days (not *during* five days).

We use *during* + noun to say when something happens (not how long):

- The resident fell asleep *during* the MR diffusion conference.

We use *while* + subject + verb:

- The resident fell asleep *while* he was attending the MR diffusion conference.

By **and** Until

By + a time (i.e., not later than; you cannot use *until* with this meaning):

- I mailed the article on carotid dissection today, so they should receive it *by* Tuesday.

Until can be used to say how long a situation continues:

- Let's wait *until* the patient gets better.

When you are talking about the past, you can use *by the time*:

- *By the time* they got to the hotel the congress had already started.

In/At/On

We use *in* as in the following examples:

- *In* a room
- *In* a building
- *In* a town/*in* a country (Dr. Vida works *in* Cordoba.)
- *In* the water/ocean/river
- *In* a row
- *In* the hospital

We use *at* as in the following examples:

- *At* the bus stop
- *At* the door/window
- *At* the top/bottom
- *At* the airport
- *At* work
- *At* sea
- *At* an event (I saw Dr. Jules *at* the residents' party.)

We use *on* as in the following examples:
- *On* the ceiling
- *On* the floor
- *On* the wall
- *On* a page
- *On* your nose
- *On* a farm

In or At?

- We say *in the corner of a room*, but *at the corner of a street*.

- We say *in* or *at* college/school. Use *at* when you are thinking of the college/school as a place or when you give the name of the college/school:
  - Thomas will be *in* college for three more years.
  - He studied medicine *at* Harvard Medical School.

- With buildings, you can use *in* or *at*.

- *Arrive.* We say:
  - *Arrive in* a country or town (Dr. Vida *arrived in* Boston yesterday.)
  - *Arrive at* other places (Dr. Vida *arrived at* the airport a few minutes ago.)
  - But: *arrive home* (Dr. Vida *arrived home* late after sending the article to AJR.)

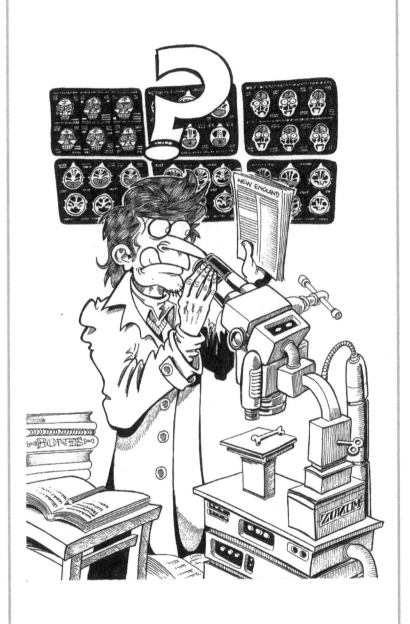

Unit III Scientific Literature: Writing an Article

This chapter is not intended to be a "Guide for Authors" such as those that you can find in any journal. Our main advice is: do not write the paper first in your own language and then translate it into English; instead, do it in English directly.

Preliminary Work

When you have a subject that you want to report, first of all you need to look up references. You can refer to the *Index Medicus* (http://www.ncbi.nlm.nih.gov/entrez/query.fcgi?db=PubMed) to search for articles. Once you have found them, read them thoroughly and underline those sentences or paragraphs that you think you might quote in your article.

Our advice is not to write the paper in your own language and then translate it into English; instead, write in English directly. In order to do so, pick up, either out of these references, or out of the journal in which you want your work to be published, the article that you find closest to the type of study that you want to report.

Although you must follow the instructions of the journal to which you want to send the paper, here we use a standard form that may be adequate for most of them. In each section, we give you a few examples just to show how you can get them from other articles.

Article Header

Title

The title of the article should be concise but informative. Put a lot of thought into the title of your article.

Abstract

An abstract of 150–250 words (it depends on the journal) must be submitted with each manuscript. Remember that an abstract is a synopsis, *not* an introduction to the article.

The abstract should answer the question: "What should readers know after reading this article."

Most journals require that the abstract is divided into four paragraphs with the following headings.

Objective

To state the purposes of the study or investigation; the hypothesis being tested or the procedure being evaluated.

Notice that very often you may construct the sentence beginning with an infinitive tense:

- *To evaluate* the impact of false-positive marks from computer-aided detection (CAD) in screening mammography.
- *To present* our experience of AVM embolization.
- *To study* the diagnostic value of SPECT for multiple myeloma (MM).
- *To assess* bone marrow angiogenesis in patients with acute myeloid leukemia (AML) by iron oxide-enhanced MRI.
- *To compare* the image acquisition time for digital versus film-screen imaging for screening mammography in a hard copy interpretation environment.
- *To determine* the prevalence of stenoses in dysfunctional autogenous hemodialysis fistulas, patency following angioplasty and to identify predictors of this patency.
- *To develop* an efficient and fully unsupervised method to quantitatively assess myocardial contraction from 4D-tagged MR sequences.
- *To investigate* the prognostic value of FDG PET uptake parameters in patients who undergo an R0 resection for carcinoma of the lung.
- *To ascertain* recent trends in imaging workload among the various medical specialties.
- *To describe* the clinical presentation, sonographic diagnosis and radiological treatment of uterine AVMs.
- *To assess* the usefulness of three-dimensional (3D) gadolinium-enhanced MR urethrography and virtual MR urethroscopy in the evaluation of urethral pathologies.
- *To establish* ..., *To perform* ..., *To study* ..., *To design* ..., *To analyze* ..., *To test* ..., *To define* ..., *To illustrate* ...

You can also begin with: "The aim/purpose/objective/goal of this study was to …":

- *The aim of this study was to* determine the prognostic importance of small hypoattenuating hepatic lesions on contrast-enhanced CT in patients with breast cancer.
- *The purpose of this study was to* compare feasibility and precision of renal artery stent placement using two different MR guidance techniques.
- *The objective of this study was to* determine whether acute myocardial infarction (MI) can be diagnosed on contrast-enhanced helical chest CT.

You may give some background and then state what you have done.

- *Autoimmune pancreatitis is a new clinical entity which frequently mimics pancreatic carcinoma, resulting in unnecessary radical surgery of the pancreas. The purpose of this study was to describe radiologic findings of autoimmune pancreatitis.*
- *Myocardial fibrosis is known to occur in patients with hypertrophic cardiomyopathy (HCM) and to be associated with myocardial dysfunction. This study was designed to clarify the relation between myocardial fibrosis demonstrated by gadolinium-enhanced magnetic resonance imaging (Gd-MRI) and procollagen peptides or cytokines.*
- *… We hypothesized that …*
- *… We compared …*
- *… We investigated …*

Materials and Methods

Briefly state what was done and what materials were used, including the number of subjects. Also include the methods used to assess the data and to control bias.

- N *patients with … were included.*
- N *patients with … were excluded.*
- N *patients known to have/suspected of having …*
- *… was performed in* N *patients with …*
- N *patients underwent …*
- *Quantitative/Qualitative analyses were performed by …*

- *Patients were followed clinically for ... months/years.*
- *We examined the effects of iodinated IV contrast on blood pressure, heart rate and renal function after a CT scan in 14 healthy young volunteers.*

Results

Provide the findings of the study, including indicators of statistical significance. Include actual numbers, as well as percentages.

- *24 lesions were found. 15 (62.5%) were isointense, 4 (16.5%) hyperintense and 5 (21%) hypointense in the sequences acquired 90 minutes after the administration of the liver-specific paramagnetic contrast agent. 13 lesions (54%) presented an enhancing peripheral ring. All 6 patients also studied with 3D GE T1-weighted thinner slices (thickness 2.5 mm) had an enhancing peripheral ring (100%).*
- *Hemidiaphragmatic elevation on plain radiographs and fluoroscopic paradoxical movement of the diaphragm after transarterial chemoembolization (TACE) via the inferior phrenic artery (IPA) were observed in 6/15 patients (40%) and 7/15 patients (46.7%), respectively. Vital capacity decreased from the pre-TACE measurements (% of predictive value) of 88.80+19.95 to 82.60+19.33 after TACE (p=0.05). No significant correlation was noted between the dosage of chemoembolic agents and the presence or absence of paradoxical diaphragmatic movement or vital capacity lung.*
- *Twelve patients had acute myocardial infarction (AMI) and nine patients acute myocarditis (AM). All AMI but one displayed a territorial early subendocardial defect with corresponding delayed enhancement. All AMI displayed stenosis of at least the corresponding coronary artery. All AM but one displayed normal first-pass enhancement patterns and focal or diffuse nonterritorial nonsubendocardial delayed enhancement with normal coronary arteries in all cases.*

Conclusion

Summarize in one or two sentences the conclusion(s) made on the basis of the findings. It should emphasize new and important aspects of the study or observations.

- *Multi-detector row CT is an effective tool for depicting orthopedic hardware complications.*
- *Contrast enhancement characteristics of breast cancer are significantly affected by contrast injection rate. It is critical to incorporate contrast injection rate into pharmacokinetic modeling for accurate characterization of breast cancer.*
- *Contrast-enhanced color Doppler imaging demonstrated an overall accuracy of 100% for the detection of crossing vessels at the obstructed UPJ. This technique showed comparable results to CT and MRI and therefore provides accurate information for the detection of vessels crossing at the obstructed UPJ.*
- *US is moderately accurate in the diagnosis of substantial fatty atrophy of the supraspinatus or infraspinatus muscles.*
- *The study data demonstrate ..., Preliminary findings indicate ..., Results suggest ...*

Keywords

Below the abstract you should provide, and identify as such, three to ten keywords or short phrases that will assist indexers in cross-indexing the article and may be published with the abstract. The terms used should be from the Medical Subject Headings list of the Index Medicus (http://www.nlm.nih.gov/mesh/meshhome.html).

Main Text

The text of observational and experimental articles is usually (but not necessarily) divided into sections with the headings *Introduction, Methods, Results,* and *Discussion.* Long articles may need subheadings within some sections (especially the Results and Discussion sections) to clarify their content. Other types of articles, such as Case Reports, Reviews, and Editorials, are likely to need other formats. You should consult individual journals for further guidance.

Avoid using abbreviations. When used, abbreviations should be spelled out the first time a term is given in the text, for example *magnetic resonance imaging (MRI).*

Introduction

The text should begin with an Introduction that conveys the nature and purpose of the work, and quotes the relevant literature. Give only strictly pertinent background information necessary for understanding why the topic is important and references that inform the reader as to why you undertook your study. Do not review the literature extensively. The final paragraph should clearly state the hypothesis or purpose of your study. Brevity and focus are important.

Materials and Methods

Details of clinical and technical procedures should follow the Introduction.

Describe your selection of the observational or experimental subjects (patients or laboratory animals, including controls) clearly. Identify the age, sex, and other important characteristics of the subjects. Because the relevance of such variables as age, sex, and ethnicity to the object of research is not always clear, authors should explicitly justify them when they are included in a study report. The guiding principle should be clarity about how and why a study was done in a particular way. For example, authors should explain why only subjects of certain ages were included or why women were excluded. You should avoid terms such as "race", which lack precise biological meaning, and use alternative concepts such as "ethnicity" or "ethnic group" instead. You should also specify carefully what the descriptors mean, and say exactly how the data were collected (for example, what terms were used in survey forms, whether the data were self-reported or assigned by others, etc.).

- *Our study population was selected from ...*
- *N patients underwent ...*
- *N consecutive patients ...*
- *N patients with proven ...*
- *Patients were followed clinically ...*
- *N patients with ... were examined before and during ...*
- *N patients with known or suspected ... were prospectively enrolled in this study.*
- *More than N patients presenting with ... were examined with ... over a period of N months.*
- *N patients were prospectively enrolled between ... (date) and ... (date).*
- *N patients (N men, N women; age range N–N years; mean N.N years).*
- *In total, 140 patients, aged 30–50 years (mean 40 years), all with severe acute pancreatitis fulfilling Ramson criteria, were included in the study.*
- *Patients undergoing elective coronary arteriography for evaluation of chest pain were considered eligible if angiography documented ...*

Identify the methods, instrumentation (trade names and manufacturer's name and location in parentheses), and procedures in sufficient detail to allow other workers to reproduce your study. Identify precisely all drugs and chemicals used, including generic name(s), dose(s), and route(s) of administration.

- *MR imaging was performed with a 1.5-T system (Vision; Siemens, Erlangen, Germany).*
- *The US-guided biopsy procedures were performed using model RT 3000 equipment (GE Medical Systems, Milwaukee, Wis.) with either a 3.5- or a 5-MHz sector transducer combined with a needle guide or a 5-MHz linear-array transducer with a free-hand technique.*
- *Automatic high-speed core biopsy equipment (Biopty instrument and Biopty-Cut needles; Bard Urological, Covington, Ga.) was used.*
- *After baseline PET investigation, 40 mg of fluvastatin (Cranoc, Astra) was administered once daily.*
- *Dynamic PET measurements were performed with a whole-body scanner (CTI/ECAT 951R/31; Siemens/CTI). After a transmission scan for attenuation correction, 20 mCi of ^{13}N-labeled ammonia was administered as a bolus over 30 seconds by an infusion pump. The dynamic PET data acquisition consisted of varying frame durations (12×10 seconds, 6×30 seconds, and 3×300 seconds). For the stress study, adenosine was infused at a dose of 0.14 mg$\cdot$kg$^{-1}\cdot$min^{-1} over 5 minutes. ^{13}N-labeled ammonia was administered in a similar fashion as in the baseline study during the third minute of the adenosine infusion.*

It is essential that you state the manner by which studies were evaluated: independent readings, consensus readings, blinded or unblinded to other information, time sequencing between readings of several studies of the same patient or animal to eliminate recall bias, random ordering of studies. It should be clear as to the retrospective or prospective nature of your study.

- *Entry/inclusion criteria included ...*
- *These criteria had to be met: ...*
- *Patients with ... were not included.*
- *Further investigations, including ... and ..., were also performed.*
- *We prospectively studied N patients with ...*
- *The reviews were not blinded to the presence of ...*
- *The following patient inclusion criteria were used: age between 16 and 50 years and closed epiphyses, ACL injury of one knee that required surgical replacement with a bone-to-patellar tendon-to-bone autograft, and signed informed consent with agreement to attend follow-up visits. The following exclusion criteria were used: additional ligament laxities*

> *with a grade higher than 2 (according to the European classification of frontal laxity) in the affected knee, ...*
> - *Two skeletal radiologists (O.J., C.V.) in consensus studied the following parameters on successive MR images ...*
> - *Both the interventional cardiologists and echocardiographers who performed the study and evaluated the results were blinded to drug administration.*
> - *Histologic samples were evaluated in a blinded manner by one of the authors and an outside expert in rodent liver pathology.*

Give references to established methods, including statistical methods that have been published but are not well known; describe new or substantially modified methods and give reasons for using these techniques, and evaluate their limitations. Identify precisely all drugs and chemicals used, including generic name(s), dose(s), and route(s) of administration. Do no use a drug's trade name unless it is directly relevant.

> - *The imaging protocol included ...*
> - *To assess objectively the severity of acute pancreatitis, all patients were scored using the Balthazar criteria (10).*
> - *The stereotactic device used for breast biopsy has been described elsewhere (12); it consists of a ...*
> - *Gut permeability was measured in isolated intestinal segments as described previously (2).*

Statistics

Describe statistical methods with enough detail to enable a knowledgeable reader with access to the original data to verify the reported results. Put a general description of methods in the Methods section. When data are summarized in the Results section, specify the statistical methods used to analyze them:

> - *The statistical significance of differences was calculated with Fisher's exact test.*
> - *The probability of ... was calculated using the Kaplan-Meier method.*
> - *To test for statistical significance, ...*
> - *Statistical analyses were performed with ... and ... tests.*
> - *The levels of significance are indicated by P values.*
> - *Interobserver agreement was quantified by using k statistics.*
> - *All P values of less than 0.05 were considered to indicate statistical significance.*

- *Univariate and multivariate Cox proportional hazards regression models were used.*
- *The v^2-test was used for group comparison. Descriptive values of variables are expressed as means and percentages.*
- *We adjusted RRs for age (5-year categories) and used the Mantel extension test to test for linear trends. To adjust for other risk factors, we used multiple logistic regression.*

Give details about randomization:

- *They were selected consecutively by one physician between February 1999 and June 2000.*
- *This study was conducted prospectively during a period of 30 months from March 1998 to August 2000. We enrolled 29 consecutive patients who had ...*

Specify any general-use computer programs used:

- *All statistical analyses were performed with SAS software (SAS Institute, Cary, N.C.).*
- *The statistical analyses were performed using a software package (SPSS for Windows, release 8.0; SPSS, Chicago, Ill.).*

Results

Present your results in logical sequence in the text, along with tables, and illustrations. Do not repeat in the text all the data in the tables or illustrations; emphasize or summarize only important observations. Avoid non-technical uses of technical terms in statistics, such as "random" (which implies a randomizing device), "normal", "significant", "correlations", and "sample". Define statistical terms, abbreviations, and most symbols:

- *Statistically significant differences were shown for both X and X.*
- *Significant correlation was found between X and X.*
- *Results are expressed as means ±SD.*
- *All the abnormalities in our patient population were identified on the prospective clinical interpretation.*
- *The abnormalities were correctly characterized in 14 patients and incorrectly in ...*
- *The preoperative and operative characteristics of these patients are listed in Table 1.*

- *The results of the US-guided core-needle pleural biopsies are shown in Table 1.*
- *The clinical findings are summarized in Table 1.*

Report any complication:

- *Two minor complications were encountered. After the second procedure, one patient had a slight hemoptysis that did not require treatment, and one patient had local chest pain for about 1 hour after a puncture in the supraclavicular region. Pneumothorax was never encountered.*
- *Among the 11,101 patients, there were 373 in-hospital deaths (3.4%), 204 intraoperative/postoperative CVAs (1.8%), 353 patients with post-operative bleeding events (3.2%), and 142 patients with sternal wound infections (1.3%).*

Give numbers of observations. Report losses to observation (such as drop-outs from a clinical trial):

- *The final study cohort consisted of ...*
- *Of the 961 patients included in this study, 69 were reported to have died (including 3 deaths identified through the NDI), and 789 patients were interviewed (Figure 1). For 81 surviving patients, information was obtained from another source. Twenty-two patients (2.3%) could not be contacted and were not included in the analyses because information on nonfatal events was not available.*

Discussion

Within this section, use ample subheadings. Emphasize the new and important aspects of the study and the conclusions that follow from them. Do not repeat in detail data or other material given in the Introduction or the Results sections. Include in the Discussion section the implications of the findings and their limitations, including implications for future research. Relate the observations to other relevant studies.

Link the conclusions with the goals of the study, but avoid unqualified statements and conclusions not completely supported by the data. In particular, avoid making statements on economic benefits and costs unless the report includes economic data and analyses. Avoid claiming priority and alluding to work that has not been completed. State new hypotheses when warranted, but clearly label them as such. Recommendations, when appropriate, may be included.

- *In conclusion, ...*
- *In summary, ...*
- *This study demonstrates that ...*
- *This study found that ...*
- *This study highlights ...*
- *Another finding of our study is ...*
- *One limitation of our study was ...*
- *Other methodological limitations of this study ...*
- *Our results support ...*
- *Further research is needed to elucidate ...*
- *However, the limited case number warrants a more comprehensive study to confirm these findings and to assess the comparative predictive value of relative lung volume versus LHR.*
- *Some follow-up is probably appropriate for these patients.*
- *Further research is needed when endoluminal surface coil technology is available.*

Acknowledgments

List all contributors who do not meet the criteria for authorship, such as a person who provided purely technical help, writing assistance, or a department chair who provided only general support. Financial and material support should also be acknowledged.

People who have contributed materially to the paper but whose contributions do not justify authorship may be listed under a heading such as "clinical investigators" or "participating investigators," and their function or contribution should be described: for example, "served as scientific advisors," "critically reviewed the study proposal," "collected data," or "provided and cared for study patients."

Because readers may infer their endorsement of the data and conclusions, everybody must have given written permission to be acknowledged.

- *The authors express their gratitude to ... for their excellent technical support.*
- *The authors thank Wei J. Chen, MD, ScD, Institute of Epidemiology, College of Public Health, National Taiwan University, Taipei, for the analysis of the statistics and his help in the evaluation of the data. The authors also thank Pan C. Yang, MD, PhD, Department of Internal Medicine, and Keh S. Tsai, MD, PhD, Department of Laboratory Medicine, National Taiwan University, Medical College and Hospital, Taipei, for the inspiration and discussion of the research idea of this study. We also thank Ling C. Shen for her assistance in preparing the manuscript.*

References

References should be numbered consecutively in the order in which they are first mentioned in the text. Identify references in text, tables, and legends by Arabic numerals in parentheses (some journals require superscript Arabic numbers). References cited only in tables or figure legends should be numbered in accordance with the sequence established by the first citation in the text of the particular table or figure.

- *Clinically, resting thallium-201 (^{201}Tl) single photon emission computed tomography (SPECT) has been widely used to evaluate myocardial viability in patients with chronic coronary arterial disease and acute myocardial infarction (8–16).*
- *In addition, we have documented a number of other parameters previously shown to exhibit diurnal variation, including an assessment of sympathetic activity, as well as inflammatory markers recently shown to relate to endothelial function.[14]*

Use the style of the examples below, which are based on the formats used by the NLM in *Index Medicus*. The titles of journals should be abbreviated according to the style used in *Index Medicus*. Consult the *List of Journals Indexed in Index Medicus*, published annually as a separate publication by the library and as a list in the January issue of *Index Medicus*. The list can also be obtained through the library's website (http://www.nlm.nih.gov).

Avoid using abstracts as references. References to papers accepted but not yet published should be designated as "in press" or "forthcoming"; authors should obtain written permission to cite such papers as well as verification that they have been accepted for publication. Information from articles submitted but not accepted should be cited in the text as "unpublished observations" with written permission from the source.

Avoid citing a "personal communication" unless it provides essential information not available from a public source, in which case the name of the person and date of communication should be cited in parentheses in the text. For scientific articles, authors should obtain written permission and confirmation of accuracy from the source of a personal communication.

The references must be verified by the author(s) against the original documents.

The Uniform Requirements style (the Vancouver style) is based largely on an ANSI standard style adapted by the NLM for its databases. Notes have been added where Vancouver style differs from the style now used by NLM.

Articles in Journals

Standard Journal Article

List the first six authors followed by et al. (*Note*: NLM now lists up through 25 authors; if there are more than 25 authors, NLM lists the first 24, then the last author, then et al.)

> *Theodorou SJ, Theodorou DJ, Schweitzer ME, Kakitsubata Y, Resnick D. Magnetic resonance imaging of para-acetabular insufficiency fractures in patients with malignancy. Clin Radiol 2006 Feb; 61(2):181–190.*

As an option, if a journal carries continuous pagination throughout a volume (as many medical journals do) the month and issue number may be omitted. (*Note*: for consistency, the option is used throughout the examples in Uniform Requirements. NLM does not use the option.)

> *Theodorou SJ, Theodorou DJ, Schweitzer ME, Kakitsubata Y, Resnick D. Magnetic resonance imaging of para-acetabular insufficiency fractures in patients with malignancy. Clin Radiol 2006; 61:181–190.*

Organization as Author

> *The Evidence-based Radiology Working Group. Evidence-based radiology: a new approach to the practice of radiology. Radiology 2001; 220:566–575.*

No Author Given

> *Cancer in South Africa [editorial]. S Afr Med J 1994; 84:15.*

Article Not In English

(Note: NLM translates the title to English, encloses the translation in square brackets, and adds an abbreviated language designator.)

> *Zangos S, Mack MG, Straub R, et al. [Transarterial chemoembolization (TACE) of liver metastases: a palliative therapeutic approach]. Radiologie 2001:41 (1):84–90. German*

Volume with Supplement

Shen HM, Zhang QF. Risk assessment of nickel carcinogenicity and occupational lung cancer. Environ Health Perspect 1994; 102 Suppl 1:275–282.

Issue with Supplement

Payne DK, Sullivan MD, Massie MJ. Women's psychological reactions to breast cancer. Semin Oncol 1996; 23(1 Suppl 2):89–97.
Hamm B, Staks T, Taupitz M. SHU 555A: a new superparamagnetic iron oxide contrast agent for magnetic resonance imaging. Invest Radiol 1994; 29(Suppl 2):S87–S89.

Volume with Part

Ozben T, Nacitarhan S, Tuncer N. Plasma and urine sialic acid in non-insulin dependent diabetes mellitus. Ann Clin Biochem 1995; 32(Pt 3): 303–306.

Issue with Part

Poole GH, Mills SM. One hundred consecutive cases of flap lacerations of the leg in ageing patients. N Z Med J 1994; 107(986 Pt 1):377–378.

Issue with No Volume

Turan I, Wredmark T, Fellander-Tsai L. Arthroscopic ankle arthrodesis in rheumatoid arthritis. Clin Orthop 1995; (320):110–114.

No Issue or Volume

Browell DA, Lennard TW. Immunologic status of the cancer patient and the effects of blood transfusion on antitumor responses. Curr Opin Gen Surg 1993:325–333.

Pages in Roman Numerals

Fisher GA, Sikic BI. Drug resistance in clinical oncology and hematology. Introduction. Hematol Oncol Clin North Am 1995 Apr; 9(2):xi–xii.

Type of Article Indicated as Needed

Enzensberger W, Fischer PA. Metronome in Parkinson's disease [letter]. Lancet 1996; 347:1337.
Clement J, De Bock R. Hematological complications of hantavirus nephropathy (HVN) [abstract]. Kidney Int 1992; 42:1285.

Article Containing Retraction

Garey CE, Schwarzman AL, Rise ML, Seyfried TN. Ceruloplasmin gene defect associated with epilepsy in EL mice [retraction of Garey CE, Schwarzman AL, Rise ML, Seyfried TN. In: Nat Genet 1994; 6:426–431]. Nat Genet 1995; 11:104.

Article Retracted

Liou GI, Wang M, Matragoon S. Precocious IRBP gene expression during mouse development [retracted in Invest Ophthalmol Vis Sci 1994; 35:3127]. Invest Ophthalmol Vis Sci 1994; 35:1083–8.

Article with Published Erratum

Hamlin JA, Kahn AM. Herniography in symptomatic patients following inguinal hernia repair [published erratum appears in West J Med 1995; 162:278]. West J Med 1995; 162:28–31.

Books and Other Monographs

Personal Author(s)

Helms CA. Fundamentals of skeletal radiology. 1st ed. Philadelphia: WB Saunders Company; 1992.

(Note: Previous Vancouver style incorrectly had a comma rather than a semicolon between the publisher and the date.)

Editor(s), Compiler(s) as Author

Rumack CM, Wilson SR, Charboneau JW, editors. Diagnostic ultrasound. St Louis: Mosby-Year Book; 1998.

Organization as Author and Publisher

Institute of Medicine (US). Looking at the future of the Medicaid program. Washington: The Institute; 1992.

Chapter in a Book

Levine MS. Benign tumors of the esophagus. In: Gore RM, Levine MS, editors. Textbook of gastrointestinal radiology. 2nd ed. Philadelphia, Pa: Saunders; 2000. pp. 387–402.

(Note: Previous Vancouver style had a colon rather than a p before pagination.)

Conference Proceedings

Kimura J, Shibasaki H, editors. Recent advances in clinical neurophysiology. Proceedings of the 10th International Congress of EMG and Clinical Neurophysiology; 1995 Oct 15–19; Kyoto, Japan. Amsterdam: Elsevier; 1996.

Conference Paper

Bengtsson S, Solheim BG. Enforcement of data protection, privacy and security in medical informatics. In: Lun KC, Degoulet P, Piemme TE, Rienhoff O, editors. MEDINFO 92. Proceedings of the 7th World Congress on Medical Informatics; 1992 Sep 6–10; Geneva, Switzerland. Amsterdam: North-Holland; 1992. pp. 1561–1565.

Scientific or Technical Report

Issued by funding/sponsoring agency:

Smith P, Golladay K. Payment for durable medical equipment billed during skilled nursing facility stays. Final report. Dallas (TX): Dept. of Health and Human Services (US), Office of Evaluation and Inspections; 1994 Oct. Report No.: HHSIGOEI69200860.

Issued by performing agency:

Field MJ, Tranquada RE, Feasley JC, editors. Health services research: work force and educational issues. Washington: National Academy Press; 1995. Contract No.: AHCPR282942008. Sponsored by the Agency for Health Care Policy and Research.

Dissertation

Kaplan SJ. Post-hospital home health care: the elderly's access and utilization [dissertation]. St. Louis (MO): Washington Univ.; 1995.

Patent

Larsen CE, Trip R, Johnson CR, inventors; Novoste Corporation, assignee. Methods for procedures related to the electrophysiology of the heart. US patent 5,529,067. 1995 Jun 25.

Other Published Material

Newspaper Article

Lee G. Hospitalizations tied to ozone pollution: study estimates 50,000 admissions annually. The Washington Post 1996 Jun 21; Sect. A:3 (col. 5).

Audiovisual Material

HIV+/AIDS: the facts and the future [videocassette]. St. Louis (MO): Mosby Year-Book; 1995.

Dictionary and Similar References

> Stedman's medical dictionary. 26th ed. Baltimore: Williams & Wilkins; 1995. Apraxia; pp. 119–120.

Unpublished Material

In Press

(Note: NLM prefers "forthcoming" because not all items will be printed.)

> Assessment of chest pain in the emergency room: What is the role of multidetector CT? Eur J Radiol. In press 2006.

Electronic Material

Journal Article in Electronic Format

> Morse SS. Factors in the emergence of infectious diseases. Emerg Infect Dis [serial online] 1995 Jan-Mar [cited 1996 Jun 5]; 1(1):[24 screens]. Available from: URL: http://www.cdc.gov/ncidod/EID/eid.htm.

Monograph in Electronic Format

> CDI, clinical dermatology illustrated [monograph on CD-ROM]. Reeves JRT, Maibach H. CMEA Multimedia Group, producers. 2nd ed. Version 2.0. San Diego: CMEA; 1995.

Computer File

> Hemodynamics III: the ups and downs of hemodynamics [computer program]. Version 2.2. Orlando (FL): Computerized Educational Systems; 1993.

Additional Material

Tables

All tabulated data identified as tables should be given a table number and a descriptive caption. Take care that each table is cited in numerical sequence in the text.

The presentation of data and information given in the table headings should not duplicate information already given in the text. Explain in footnotes all non-standard abbreviations used in the table.

If you need to use any table or figure from another journal, make sure you ask for permission and put a note such as:

Adapted, with permission, from reference 5.

Figures

Figures should be numbered consecutively in the order in which they are first cited in the text. Follow the "pattern" of similar illustrations of your references.

- *Figure 1. Non-enhanced CT scan shows ...*

- *Figure 2. Contrast-enhanced CT scan obtained at the level of ...*

- *Figure 3. Selective renal arteriogram shows ...*

- *Figure 4. Photograph of a fresh-cut specimen shows ...*

- *Figure 5. Photomicrograph (original magnification, ×10; hematoxylin-eosin stain) of ...*

- *Figure 6. Coronal contrast-enhanced T1-weighted MR image of ...*

- *Figure 7. Typical metastatic compression fracture in a 65-year-old man. (a) Sagittal T1-weighted MR image (400/11) shows ...*

- *Figure 6. Nasal-type extranodal NK/T-cell lymphoma involving the nasal cavity in a 42-year-old woman. Photomicrograph (original magnification, ×400; hematoxylin-eosin [H-E] stain) of a nasal mucosal biopsy specimen shows intense infiltration of atypical lymphoid cells into the vascular intima and subintima (arrow). This is a typical appearance of angiocentric invasion in which the vascular lumen (V) is nearly obstructed.*

- *Figure 7. AFX with distortion of histopathologic architecture as a consequence of intratumoral ...*

- *Figure 8. CT images obtained in a 75-year-old man with gross hematuria. (a) MIP image obtained during the compression-release excretory phase demonstrates a non-obstructing calculus (arrow) in the distal portion of the right ureter.*

Final Tips

Before you submit your article for publication check its spelling, and go over your article for words you might have omitted or typed twice, as well as words you may have misused such as using "there" instead of "their." Do not send an article with spelling or dosage errors or other medical inaccuracies. And do not expect the spell-check function on your computer to catch all your spelling mistakes.

Be accurate. Check and double-check your facts and reference citations. Even after you feel the article is finished leave it for a day or two and then go back to it. The changes you make to your article after seeing it in a new light will often be the difference between a good article and a great article.

Once you believe everything is correct, give the draft to your English teacher for a final informal editing. Do not send your first (or even second) draft to the publisher!

Do not forget to read and follow carefully the specific "Instructions for authors" of the journal in which you want your work to be published.

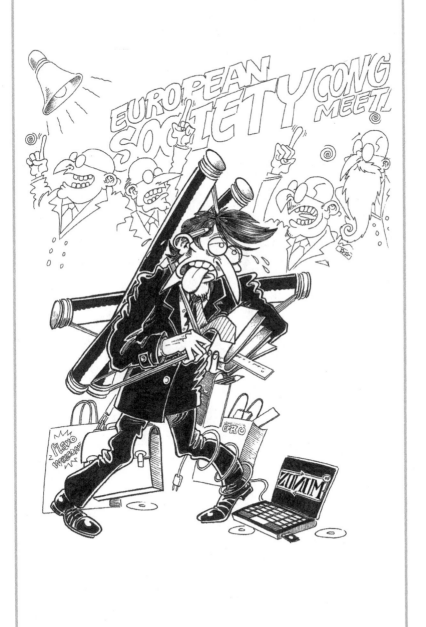

Unit IV   Letters to Editors of Radiological Journals

This unit is made up of several examples of letters sent to editors of radiological journals. Our intention is to provide you with useful tools to communicate with journal editors and reviewers in a formal manner. It is our understanding that letters to editors have quite an important, and many times overlooked, role in the fate of scientific radiological manuscripts.

Although we are not going to focus on letters from editors since they are, generally speaking, easy to understand, these letters can be divided into acceptance "under certain conditions" letters, acceptance letters, and rejection letters.

- Acceptance "under certain conditions" letters. These letters, are relatively common, and usually mean a great deal of work since the paper must be re-written.
- Acceptance letters. Congratulations! Your paper has finally been accepted and no corrections have to be made. These letters are, unfortunately, relatively uncommon, and quite easy to read. Besides, they do not need to be replied to.
- Rejection letters. There are many polite formulas of letting you know that your paper is not going to be published in a particular journal. These letters are instantly understood and since they do not need to be replied to, no time needs to be wasted on them from an idiomatic point of view.

We have divided up the letters to editors into:

- Submission letters
- Re-submission letters
- Re-configuration letters
- Letters of thanks for an invitation to publish an article in a journal
- Letters asking about the status of a paper
- Other letters

Submission Letters

Submission letters are quite easy to write since the only message to be conveyed is the type and title of the paper you are submitting and the name of the corresponding author. Many standard letters can be used for this purpose and we do not think you have to waste too much time on them since they are mere preliminary material that just needs to be sent along with the paper itself.

Your address   Date

Receiver's name and address

Dear Dr. Massa,

Please find enclosed (*N*) copies of our manuscript entitled "..." (authors ..., ..., ...), which we hereby submit for publication in the ... Journal of .... Also enclosed is a diskette with a copy of the text file in Microsoft Word for Windows (version ...).

I look forward to hearing from you.

Yours sincerely,

A. J. Merckel, MD

Re-submission Letters

Re-submission letters must thoroughly address the comments and suggestions of acceptance letters. It is in these letters where the corresponding author must let the editor know that all or at least most of the suggested changes have been made and, in doing so, the paper could be ready for publication. These letters may play quite an important role in the acceptance or rejection of a paper. Sometimes a lack of fluency in English prevents the corresponding author conveying the corrections made in the manuscript and the reasons why other suggested changes were not made.

Let's review the following example:

Dear Dr. Ho,

After a thorough revision in light of the reviewers' comments, we have decided to submit our paper "MRI evaluation of extrahepatic cholangiocarcinoma" for re-evaluation.

First of all, we would like to thank you for this second chance to present our paper for publication in your journal.

The main changes in the paper are related to your major comments:
- to improve overall image quality (including some new cases).
- to indicate what the clinical role of MRI is.
- to present our imaging diagnostic algorithm in cases of extrahepatic cholangiocarcinoma (new Tables 2 and 3).

Following your advice, we have also included changes that are in accordance with the reviewers' comments.

We hope this new version will now be suitable for publication in your journal.

Yours sincerely,

Antonio Belafonte, MD, and co-authors

Re-configuration Letters

Sometimes the paper is accepted provided its configuration is changed, i.e., from a pictorial review to a pictorial essay. Re-configuration letters are re-submission letters as well and, therefore, tend to be long.

Review this example from which we have extracted and underlined several sentences that can help you in your correspondence with journals.

"Magnetic Resonance Evaluation of focal splenic lesions" RE:01-1343

Dear Dr. Woods, (1)

We have re-configured the manuscript referenced above (2) in the form of a Pictorial Essay *following your suggestion (3)* and we have made as many changes as possible with regard to the reviewers' recommendations taking into account the *space limitation imposed by the new format of the paper (4).*

We have tried to cover all entities involving spleen focusing on their more characteristic imaging features and *giving priority to the most prevalent conditions (5).* The re-configuration of the manuscript has shortened it so drastically that we have had to rewrite it entirely and *for this reason we do not attach an annotated copy (6) – if you still consider this necessary we will include it (7).* Although tables are not permitted in Pictorial Essays, we think that the inclusion of a single table on the classification of focal splenic lesions would *"allow the reader to more easily categorize the described imaging findings"(8) as stated by reviewer no. 2 (9)* in his general remarks. The table has not been included due to the new format of the paper but *if you take our suggestion into consideration we will be pleased to add it (10).*

The major changes in our manuscript are:

1. *The title has been modified to* "Dynamic-enhanced MR imaging of focal splenic lesions" *following your recommendation (11).*
2. *We have included the technical parameters of our imaging protocol* although it has not been possible to expand the technical section *as suggested by reviewer no. 1 (12)* due to space limitation.
3. *Similarly,* the description of infectious lesions and lymphoma *could not be expanded as suggested by reviewer no. 2 due to space limitation (13).*
4. *With regard to figures (14):*
   a. We have included six new figures.
   b. *More sequences on a given lesion have been included (15),* as suggested, in figures 4, 7, 12, and 14.
   c. *The image quality of figure 5 has been improved (16).*

5. We have assigned distinct figures to different entities in most cases although the limited number of figures allowed – 15 – made it impossible to do it in all cases.

6. *With regard to comments on figures by reviewer no. 1 (17)*:
   - *Figure 4e is indeed an immediate phase postcontrast image (18).* Aortic enhancement is not well seen due to the poor contrast resolution of this image which was acquired a long time ago and was one of our first abdominal MR 3D acquisitions.
   - *Figure 6b shows a ghosting artifact due to poor breath-holding (19).*

7. *SPIO section has been erased (20)* due, again, to space limitation.

We look forward to hearing from you, (21)

Yours sincerely, (22)

John Best, MD, and co-authors (23)

1. *Dear Dr. Woods,*
   - This sentence ends with a comma rather than a semicolon.
2. *We have reconfigured the manuscript referenced above*
   - The content of the letter must be summarized in the first paragraph.
3. *... following your suggestion*
   - This is one of the commonest sentences in re-submission/re-configuration letters.
4. *... space limitation imposed by the new format of the paper*
   - Space limitation, provided the new format limits it, must be taken into consideration by both the authors and the reviewers.
5. *... giving priority to the most prevalent conditions*
   - May be a criterion for the shortening of the manuscript.
6. *... for this reason we do not attach an annotated copy*
   - Whenever you don't follow a suggestion, you must give an explanation.
7. *... if you still consider it necessary we will include it*
   - Always leave open the possibility of adding more information in further correspondence.
8. *... "allow the reader to more easily categorize the described imaging findings"*
   - You can use as an argument what was literally suggested by the reviewer by writing it in inverted commas.
9. *... as stated by reviewer no. 2*
   - This is a usual way of addressing a reviewer's comment.

10. *... if you take our suggestion into consideration we will be pleased to add it*
    - This sentence can be used whenever you want to include something which has not been requested by the reviewers.
11. *The title has been modified to ... following your recommendation.*
    - This is a usual way of addressing a reviewer's comment.
12. *We have included the technical parameters of our imaging protocol as suggested by reviewer no. 1*
    - This is a usual way of addressing a reviewer's comment.
13. *Similarly, ... could not be expanded as suggested by reviewer no. 2 due to space limitation*
    - Whenever you don't follow a suggestion, you must give an explanation.
14. *With regard to figures:*
    - Or *regarding figures, as regards figures, as for figures* (without the preposition "to").
15. *More sequences on a given lesion have been included*
    - This is a usual way of addressing a reviewer's comment.
16. *The image quality of figure 5 has been improved*
    - This is a usual way of addressing a reviewer's comment.
17. *With regard to comments on figures by reviewer no. 1:*
    - This is a usual way of addressing a reviewer's comment.
18. *Figure 4e is indeed an immediate phase postcontrast image*
    - This is a usual way of addressing a reviewer's comment.
19. *Figure 6b shows a ghosting artifact due to poor breath-holding*
    - This is a usual way of addressing a reviewer's comment.
20. *SPIO section has been erased due, again, to space limitation*
    - This is a usual way of addressing a reviewer's comment.
21. *We look forward to hearing from you,*
    - Remember that the verb following the verb "to look forward to" must be in its *-ing* form.
22. *Yours sincerely,*
    - Bear in mind that if you don't know the name of the editor you should write "Yours faithfully" instead.
23. *John Best, MD, and co-authors*
    - Although the corresponding author is the only one who signs the letter, sometimes a reference is made to the co-authors.

Letters of Thanks for an Invitation to Publish an Article in a Journal

These are simple and usually short letters in which we let the editor of a journal know how pleased we are regarding his/her invitation and how much we appreciate his/her consideration.

Your address   Date

Receiver's name and address

Dear Dr. Massa,

Thank you for the invitation to submit a manuscript on focal hepatic lesions to your journal.

Please find attached our paper which details our imaging protocol and makes a thorough revision of the literature on the subject.

I look forward to hearing from you.

Yours sincerely,

A. J. Cantona, MD

Asking About the Status of a Paper

In these letters we inquire about the situation of our article since we have not received any response from the journal. Regrettably in the academic world "no news" is not usually "good news", and many of these inquiries end up with a polite rejection letter.

Dear Dr. Ross,

As I have not received any response regarding the manuscript "MRCP of cholangiocarcinoma", I am interested in obtaining some information on the status of the paper.

Please, use the following e-mail address for further correspondence: sanzzap@seram.es

I look forward to hearing from you at your earliest convenience,

J. Sanz, MD, PhD

Other Letters

Applying for a Post

11 St Albans Road
London SW17 5TZ

17 November 2006

The Medical Staffing Officer
Brigham and Women's Hospital
18 Francis St
Boston, MA, USA

Dear Sir/Madam,

I wish to apply for the post of Consultant Radiologist as advertised in the European Journal of Radiology of 22 October.

I enclose my CV and the names of two referees as requested.

Yours faithfully,

Albert Mas, MD

Asking for Permission to Use Someone's Name as a Referee

Platero Heredia, 19
Córdoba 14012
SPAIN
17 April 2006

John G. Adams, MD
Department of Radiology
Massachusetts General Hospital
22 Beacon St
Boston, MA, USA

Dear Dr. Adams,

I am applying for a post of Consultant Radiologist at Brigham and Women's Hospital. I should be most grateful if you allow me to use your name as a referee.

Yours sincerely,

Guido Andreotti, MD

Postponing the Commencement of Duties

Gran Vía, 113
Madrid, 28004
Spain
17 November 2006

Robert H. Shaw, MD
Department of Radiology
Massachusetts General Hospital
22 Beacon St
Boston, MA, USA

Dear Dr. Shaw,

I would like to thank you for your letter of 11 February 2001 offering me the post of Consultant Cardiologist from 12 March 2001.

I am very pleased to accept the post but unfortunately I will not be able to arrive in Boston until 25 March 2001 due to personal reasons. Would it, therefore, be possible for you to postpone the commencement of my duties to 26 March 2001?

I look forward to hearing from you.

Yours sincerely,

Angela Maldini, MD

In Summary

To sum up, a few simple formal details must be recalled:

- "Dear Dr. Smith," is the usual way to begin an academic letter. Recall that after the name of the editor you must insert a comma instead of a semicolon, and continue the letter with a new paragraph.
- The usual formula "find enclosed ..." can nowadays be replaced by "find attached ..." taking into consideration that most papers are submitted via the internet.
- "I look forward to hearing from you" is a standard sentence at the end of any formal letter and you have to bear in mind, in order to avoid a usual mistake, that "to" is a preposition to be followed by a gerund rather than the infinitive particle of the verb that follows it. Do not make the usual mistake of writing "I look forward to hear from you". Similar formulas are: "I look forward to receiving your comments on ...", "Very truly yours,"
- "Your consideration is appreciated" or "Thank you for your and the reviewers' consideration" are standard sentences to be written at the end of letters to editors.
- "I look forward to receiving your feedback on ..." is a bit more casual formula commonly used in letters to editors.
- "Yours faithfully," is used when you do not know the name of the person you are writing to, whereas "sincerely,", "sincerely yours,", "yours sincerely," or "very truly yours," must be written when you address the letter to a person by name. Therefore, if the letter begins with "Dear Dr. Olsen," it must end up with "yours sincerely," and if it is addressed to the editor as such it must finish with "yours faithfully,". Don't forget that after the adverb or the pronoun you must insert a comma, rather than a period, and, then, your signature below.
- Whenever you cannot address one of the editors' suggestions explain why it was not possible in the re-submission letter so the reviewers do not waste time looking for it in the manuscript. For example:
  - *We have included the technical parameters of our imaging protocol although it has not been possible to expand the technical section as suggested by reviewer no. 1 due to space limitation.*

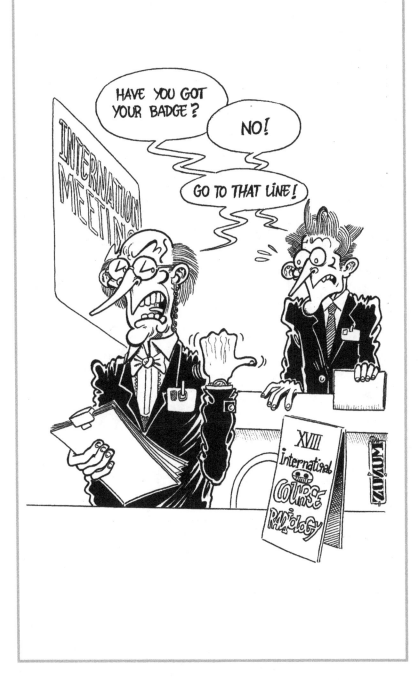

Unit V Attending an International Radiological Course

Introduction

In the following pages we take a look inside international radiological meetings. We recommend upper-intermediate English speakers to quickly go over them and intermediate English speakers to review this section thoroughly in order to become familiar with the jargon of international congresses and that of the conversational scenarios such as the airport, plane, customs, taxi, hotel checking-in, and finally the course itself that make up the usual itinerary of a radiologist attending an international course.

Most beginners do not go alone to their first courses abroad. This fact, which in principle is a relief since they do not have to cope with the idiomatic difficulties on their own, has an important drawback: most non-native English-speaking radiology residents come back to their respective countries without having uttered a single word in English. Although it may be considered quite unnatural, to speak in English with your colleagues is the only way of speaking in English during the course since over 90% of your conversations are going to be those you have with your fellow countrymen. In parties of more than two people, it's virtually impossible to do this simple exercise.

Traveling alone is the only way of speaking English during an international radiological course and, for non-native English speaking-radiologists, may be the only opportunity of keeping their English alive throughout the year. Do not waste this excellent opportunity to maintain your level of both colloquial English and radiological English.

The following anecdote illustrates the level of uncertainty young non-native English-speaking radiologists face when they attend their first international meetings. It was my first European Congress of Radiology in Vienna. When I was expecting to be attended to at the registration desk and given my congress bag, somebody asked me: "Have you got your badge?". Not knowing what badge meant I said "no" since I was unlikely to have something on me I did not even know the name of. The next sentence I heard was uttered in a very commanding voice: "Go to that line" so I obediently got into the line without knowing what on earth I was going to get from it. This was the first, but not the last, time I was in a line without having the slightest idea of what I was going to get from it. When this happens to you and you are supposed to give a lecture on, let's say, MRI of hepatocarcinoma, your desire to come back home is all that remains intact in you.

Don't let your lack of fluency in day-to-day English undermine your ability to deliver a good or even great presentation. Colloquial English and radiological English are two different worlds, and in order to be successful in the latter you must have a sound knowledge of the former.

This chapter provides you with tips and useful sentences in your itinerary to an international radiology course: airport, plane, customs, taxi, hotel checking in, and finally, the course itself. Unless you have overcome the conversational hurdles in the scenarios that come before the course, firstly, you are not going to get to the course venue and, secondly, if you do get to it you will not feel like delivering your presentation.

Most non-native English-speaking lecturers resign themselves to just giving the lecture and ... "survive", forgetting that if they do not enjoy their lecture, the audience will not enjoy it either. They think that to enjoy giving a lecture, your native tongue must be English. We strongly disagree with this point since many speakers do not enjoy their talks in their own native tongues, and it is our understanding that having a good time delivering a presentation has much more to do with your personality than with your native tongue.

Travel and Hotel Arrangements

Airport

Getting to the Airport

- How can I get to the airport?
- How soon should we be at the airport before take-off?

Checking in

- May I have your passport and flight tickets, please? Of course, here you are.
- Are you Mr. Vida? Right, I am. How do you spell it? V-I-D-A (rehearse the spelling of your last name since if it is not an English one, you are going to be asked about its spelling many times).
- Here is your boarding card. Your flight leaves from gate 43. Thank you

- You are only allowed two carry-on items. You'll have to check in that larger bag.

Questions a Passenger Might Ask

- I want to fly to London leaving this afternoon. Is there a direct flight? Is it via Zurich?
- Is it direct? Yes, it is direct/No, it is one-stop.
- Is there a stop-over? Yes, You have a stop-over in Berlin.
- How long is the stop-over? About 1 hour.
- Do I have to change planes? Yes, You have to change planes at ...
- How much carry-on luggage am I allowed?
- What weight am I allowed?
- My luggage is overweight. How much more do I need to pay?
- Is a meal served? Yes, lunch will be served during the flight.
- What time does the plane to Chicago leave?
- When does the next flight to Chicago leave?
- Can I get onto the next flight?
- Can I change my flight schedule?
- What's the departure time?
- Is the plane on time?
- What's the arrival time?
- Will I be able to make my connection?
- I have misplaced my hand luggage. Where is lost property?
- How much is it to upgrade this ticket to first class?
- I want to change the return flight date from Boston to Madrid to November 30th.
- Is it possible to purchase an open ticket?
- I have missed my flight to New York. When does the next flight leave, please?
- Can I use the ticket I have or do I need to pay for a new one?

Announcing Changes in an Airline Flight

- Our flight to Madrid has been cancelled because of snow.
- Our flight to Chicago has been delayed; however all connecting flights can be made.
- Flight number 112 to Paris has been cancelled.
- Flight number 1145 has been moved to gate B12.
- Passengers for flight number 112 to London go to gate 7. Hurry up! Our flight has been called over the loudspeaker.

At the Boarding Gate

- We will begin boarding soon.
- We are now boarding passengers in rows 24 through 36.
- May I see your boarding card?

Arrival

- Pick up your luggage at the terminal.
- Where can I find a luggage cart?
- Where is the taxi rank?
- Where is the subway stop?
- Where is the way out?

Complaining About Lost or Damaged Luggage

- My luggage is missing.
- One of my bags seems to be missing.
- My luggage is damaged.
- One of my suitcases has been lost.

Exchange Office

- Where is the exchange office?
- What is the rate for the Dollar?
- Could you change 1000 Euros into Dollars?

Customs and Immigration Control

- May I see your passport, please?
- Do you have your visa?
- What is your nationality?
- What is the purpose of your journey? The purpose of my journey is a holiday, touring, family affairs, studying ...
- How long do you plan on staying?
- Empty your pockets and put your wallet, keys, mobile phone and coins on this tray.
- Remove any metallic object you are carrying and put them on this tray.
- Open your laptop.
- Take off your shoes. Put them in this tray too.

- Do you have anything to declare? No, I don't have anything to declare.
- Do you have anything to declare? No, I only have personal effects.
- Do you have anything to declare? Yes, I am a doctor and I'm carrying some surgical instruments.
- Do you have anything to declare? Yes, I have bought six bottles of whisky and four cartons of cigarettes in the duty free.
- How much currency are you bringing into the country? I haven't got any foreign currency.
- Open your bag, please.
- I need to examine the contents of your bag.
- May I close my bag? Sure
- Please place your suitcases on the table.
- What do you have in these parcels? Some presents for my wife and kids.
- How much duty do I have to pay?
- Where is the exchange office?

During the Flight

Very few exchanges are likely during a normal flight. If you are familiar with them you will realize how fluency interferes positively with your mood. Conversely, if you need a pillow and are not able to ask for it, your self-confidence will shrink, your neck will hurt, and you will not ask for anything else during the flight. On my first flight to the States I did not know how to ask for a pillow and tried to convince myself that I did not actually need one. When I looked it up in my guide, asked for it, and the stewardess brought the pillow, I gladly and pleasantly fell asleep.

Do not let lack of fluency spoil an otherwise perfect flight.

- Is there an aisle/window seat free? (I asked for one at the check-in and they told me I should ask on board just in case there had been a cancellation.)
- Excuse me, you are in my seat. Oh! Sorry, I didn't notice.
- Fasten your seat belt, please.
- Your life-jacket is under your seat.
- Smoking is not allowed during the flight.
- Please would you bring me a blanket/pillow?
- Is there a business class seat free?
- Can I upgrade to first class on board?
- Would you like a cup of coffee/tea/a glass of soda? A glass of soda, please.

- What would you prefer, chicken or beef/fish or meat? Beef/Fish, please.
- Is there a vegetarian menu?
- Stewardess, I'm feeling bad. Do you have anything for flight-sickness? Could you bring me another sick-bag, please.
- Stewardess, I have a headache. Do you have an aspirin?
- Stewardess, this gentleman is disturbing me.

In the Taxi (*US* Cab)

Think for a moment of taking a taxi in your city. How many sentences do you suppose would be exchanged in normal, and even extraordinary, conditions? I assure you that with fewer than two dozen sentences you will solve more than ninety per cent of possible situations.

Asking Where to Get a Taxi

- Where is the nearest taxi rank?
- Where can I get a taxi?

Basic Instructions

- Hi, take me downtown/to the Sheraton hotel, please.
- Please would you take me to the Airport?
- It is rush hour, I don't go to the airport.
- Sorry, I am not on duty.
- It will cost you double fare to leave the city.
- I need to go to the Convention Center.
- Which way do you want me to take you, via Fifth or Seventh Avenue? Either one would be OK.
- Is there any surcharge to the airport?

Concerning Speed in a Taxi

- To downtown as quick as you can.
- Are you in a hurry? Yes, I'm in a hurry.
- I'm late; please hurry.
- Slow down!
- Do you have to drive so fast? There is no need to hurry. I am not in a rush at all.

Concerning Smoking in a Taxi

- Would you mind putting your cigarette out?
- Would you mind not smoking, please?

Asking to Stop and Wait

- Stop at number 112, please.
- Which side of the street?
- Do you want me to drop you at the door?
- Pull over, I'll be back in a minute.
- Please, wait here a minute.
- Stop here.

Concerning the Temperature in a Taxi

- Would you please wind your window up? It's a bit cold.
- Could you turn the heat up/down/on/off?
- Could you turn the air conditioning on/off?
- Is the air conditioning/heating on?

Payment

- How much is it?
- How much do I owe you?
- Is the tip included?
- Do you have change for a twenty/fifty (dollar bill)? Sorry, I don't (have any change).
- Keep the change.
- Would you give me a receipt?
- I need a receipt, please.
- I think that is too expensive.
- They have never charged me this before. Give me a receipt, please. I think I'll make a complaint.
- Can I pay by credit card? Sure, swipe your card here.

At the Hotel

Checking In

- May I help you?
- Hello, I have reserved a room under the name of Dr. Viamonte.
- For how many people? Two, my wife and me.
- Do you need my ID?
- Do you need my credit card?
- How long will you be staying? We are staying for a week.
- You will have to wait until your room is ready.
- Here is your key.
- Enjoy your stay. Thank you.
- Is there anybody who can help me with my bags?
- Do you need a bellboy? Yes, please.
- I'll have someone bring your luggage up.

Preferences

- Can you double-check that we have a double room with a view of the beach/city ...?
- I would like a room at the front/at the rear.
- I would like the quietest room you have.
- I would like a non-smoking room.
- I would like a suite.
- How many beds? I want a double bed/a single bed.
- I asked for two single beds.
- I'd like a king-sized bed.
- I'd like a queen-sized bed.
- We will need a crib for the baby.
- Are all of your rooms en suite? Yes, all of our rooms have a bath or shower.
- Is breakfast included?
- Does the hotel have a car park?
- Do you have a car park nearby?

The Stay

- Can you give me a wake-up call at seven each morning?
- There is no hot water. Would you please send someone to fix it?
- The TV is not working properly. Would you please send someone to fix it?

- The bathtub has no plug. Would you please send someone up with one.
- The people in the room next to mine are making a racket. Would you please tell them to keep it down?
- I want to change my room. It's too noisy.
- What time does breakfast start?
- How can I get to the city center?
- Can we change Euros into Dollars?
- Could you recommend a good restaurant near to the hotel?
- Could you recommend a good restaurant?
- Would you give me the number for room service?
- I will have a cheese omelet, a ham sandwich and an orange juice.
- Are there vending machines available?
- Do you have a fax machine available?
- Do you serve meals?
- Is there a pool/restaurant ...?
- How do I get room service?
- Is there wireless/internet connection?
- The sink is clogged.
- The toilet is running.
- The toilet is leaking.
- My toilet overflowed!
- The toilet doesn't flush.
- The bath is leaking.
- My bathroom is flooded.
- The bath faucets (*UK* taps) drip day and night.
- The water is rust-colored.
- The pipes are always banging.
- The water is too hot.
- The water is never hot enough.
- I don't have any hot water.

Checking Out

- How much is it?
- Do you accept credit cards?
- Can I pay in Dollars/Euros?
- I'd like a receipt, please.
- What time is checkout? Checkout is at 11 a.m.
- I would like to check out.
- Is there a penalty for late checkout?
- Please would you have my luggage brought down.
- Would you please call me a taxi?
- How far is the nearest bus stop/subway station?

Complaints

- Excuse me, there is a mistake on the receipt:
- I have had only one breakfast.
- I thought breakfast was included.
- I have been in a single room.
- Have you got a complaints book?
- Please would you give me my car keys?
- Is there anybody here who can help me with my luggage?

Course Example

General Information

By way of example let's review some general information concerning a course program, focusing on those terms that may not be known by beginners.

Language

The official language of the course will be English.

Dress Code

Formal dress is required for the Opening Ceremony and for the Social Dinner. Casual wear is acceptable for all other events and occasions (although formal dress is customary for lecturers).

Commercial Exhibition

Participants will have the opportunity to visit representatives from pharmaceutical, diagnostic and equipment companies, and publishers at their stands to discuss new developments and receive up-to-date product information.

Although most beginners don't talk to salespeople due to their lack of fluency in English, talking to salespeople in commercial stands is a good way to practice radiological English and, by the same token, receive up-to-date information on equipment and devices you currently use, or will use in the future, at your institution.

Disclosure Statements

To avoid commercial bias, speakers have to report whether they have significant relationships with industry or not.

As far as commercial relationships with industry are concerned there are three types of speakers:

1. Speakers (spouses/partners, and planners) who have no reported significant relationships with industry.
2. Speakers who have reported receiving something of "value" from a company whose product is related to the content of their presentations.
3. Speakers who have not provided information about their relationship with industry.

Faculty

Name and current posts of the speakers:

- Russel J. Curtin, MD. Staff Radiologist. Division of Neuroradiology, Beath Israel Deaconess Medical Center, Boston, MA

Guest Faculty

Name and current posts of speakers coming from institutions other than those organizing the course:

- Fergus B Schwartz, Professor of Radiology and Otolaryngology, Head and Neck Surgery, New York School of Medicine; New York University Medical Center, New York, NY

How to Reach ...

Arrival by plane

The international airport is situated about 25 kilometers outside the city. To reach the city center you can use the:

- City airport train. Every half-hour. Non-stop. 18 minutes from the airport direct to downtown, and from downtown direct to the airport. Fare: single, EUR 10; return, EUR 18.
- Regional railway, line 6. Travel time: 36 minutes. Frequency: every 30 minutes. Fare: single, EUR 12; return, EUR 20. Get off at "Charles Square". From there use the underground line "U7" to "Park Street".
- Bus. International Airport to ... Charles Square. Travel time: 25 minutes. Fare: EUR 8.

- Taxi. There is a taxi rank to the south of the arrival hall. A taxi to the city center costs around EUR 45 (depending on traffic).

Arrival by Train
For detailed information about the timetable you can call ...

At the railway station you can use the underground to reach the city.

Congress venue (where the course is to be held, e.g., hotel, university, convention center ...):

Continental Hotel
32 Park Street, 23089 ...
Phone: .../Fax: ...
E-mail: continentalhotel@hhs.com

To reach the venue from the city centre (Charles Square) take the U1 underground line (green). Leave the train at Park Street and take the exit marked Continental Hotel. Traveling time: approximately 10 minutes.

Financial Matters

The common European currency is the Euro.

Weather

The weather in ... in December is usually cold with occasional snow. The daytime temperatures normally range from –5° to +5°C

Registration

Generally you will have been registered beforehand and you will not have to register at the course's registration counter. If you do have to register at the congress venue, the following are some of the most usual exchanges that may take place during registration:

Radiologist:	May I have a registration form, please?
Course attendant:	Do you want me to fill it out (*UK* fill it in) for you? Are you a radiologist? Are you an ECR member? Are you attending the full course?
Radiology resident/ radiographer:	No. I'm a radiology resident (radiographer/ technologist)
Course attendant:	Can I see your chairman's confirmation letter?

Radiology resident/ radiographer:	I was told it was faxed last week. Would you check that, please?
Radiologist:	I'll pay by cash/credit card. Charge it to my credit card. Would you make out an invoice?
Course attendant:	Do you need an invoice? Do you want me to draw up an invoice?
Radiologist:	Where should I get my badge?
Course attendant:	Join that line.

Registration fees and deadlines

	Until 1 September 2005	Until 13 November 2006	After 13 November 2006
Full fee member	€ 230.-	€ 330.-	€ 450.-
Full fee non-member	€ 420.-	€ 540.-	€ 650.-
Resident member*	€ 150.-	€ 190.-	€ 260.-
Resident non-member*	€ 250.-	€ 310.-	€ 440.-
Radiographer*	€ 100.-	€ 140.-	€ 180.-
Hospital administrator*	€ 100.-	€ 140.-	€ 180.-
Single-day ticket	On-site only	On-site only	€ 240.-
Single half-day ticket (Tuesday only)	On-site only	On-site only	€ 80.-
Weekend ticket (Saturday 07:00 to Sunday 18:00)	On-site only	On-site only	€ 360.-
Industry day ticket	On-site only	On-site only	€ 90.-
Student**	On-site only	On-site only	!Free of charge!
Radiographer			€ 120.-
Full fee member			€ 180.-
Full fee non-member			€ 300.-

Course Planning

The basic idea whenever you attend an international radiology course is that you must rehearse beforehand those situations that are inevitably going to happen and, in so doing, you will keep to a minimum embarrassing situations catching you off-guard. If only I had rehearsed (at home!) the meaning of the word "badge", I wouldn't have been caught by surprise on my first course abroad. Just a few words, set phrases, and collocations must be known in a radiological course environment and we can assure

Table 1. Course plan

	8:30	10:30	12:15	14:00	16:00
Dec 4	Special focus session Categorical courses Refresher courses	State-of-the-art Scientific sessions Workshops Satellite symposium	Opening ceremony Inauguration lecture	Scientific sessions Satellite symposium	Special focus session Categorical courses Refresher courses Adjourn
Dec 5	Special focus session Categorical courses Refresher courses	... meets Italy Workshops	Honorary lecture	Scientific sessions Workshops	Special focus sessions Categorical courses Refresher courses Adjourn
Dec 6	Special focus session Categorical courses Refresher courses	... meets Hungary Workshops Satellite symposium	Honorary lecture	Image interpretation session	Special focus sessions Categorical courses Refresher courses Adjourn
Dec 7	Special focus session Categorical courses Refresher courses	State-of-the-art Workshops Scientific sessions	Honorary lecture	... meets Japan Scientific sessions	Special focus sessions Categorical courses Refresher courses Adjourn
Dec 8	Special focus session Categorical courses Refresher courses	Workshops Scientific sessions	Closing ceremony		

you that knowing them will give you the confidence needed to make your participation in the course a personal success.

The first piece of advice is: read the program of the course thoroughly and look up in the dictionary or ask your more experienced colleagues about the words and concepts you don't know. Since program is available before the course starts, go over it at home; you don't need to read the scientific program at the course's venue.

"Adjourn" is one of those typical program terms with which one gets familiar once the session is "adjourned". Although many could think that most terms are going to be integrated and understood by their context, our intention is to go over those "insignificant" terms that may prevent you from optimizing your time at the course.

An example of a course plan is presented in Table 1. The course plan may contain the following elements:

- *Satellite symposia*: Scientific events sponsored by pharmaceutical firms where new drugs (mainly contrast media), techniques or devices are presented to the radiological community.
- *Plenary sessions*: These events take place usually at midday gathering all participants around outstanding members of the radiological community.
- *Cases of the day*: A number of radiological cases covering different sections of radiology. Participants can submit their diagnosis.
- *Categorical courses*: An important radiological subject is discussed focusing on the needs of general radiologists.
- *Refresher courses*: A concrete topic is reviewed in depth by experts in that particular field.
- *"... meets" sessions*: The purpose of these sessions is to forge closer ties between some invited countries and the congress. There are dedicated sessions for the radiological communities of these nations to demonstrate the excellence of radiology in their countries to congress attendees.
- *Special focus session*: The aim of a special focus session is to deal with a relevant "hot topic", presented in such a way as to promote debate between the panelists and the audience.
- *Image interpretation session*: Two panels of distinguished radiologists share their radiological knowledge with the audience while facing unknown cases.
- *Scientific session*: The Scientific Committee selects, from all the abstracts submitted, the most outstanding basic and clinical research work, and invites the authors to make a presentation of their methods and conclusions (usually not longer than 10 to 15 minutes). A round of questions and/or comments is usually permitted.
- *Adjourn:* Close (break or recess) at the end of a session.

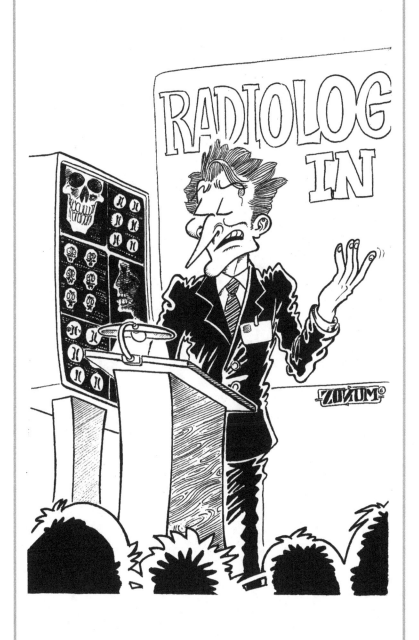

Unit VI   Giving a Radiological Talk

International radiological conferences are in a universe all of their own. In this universe, attendees and speakers come from many different countries with their own cultures and consequently their own habits in terms of behavior and public speaking. However, most speakers set aside, at least partially, their cultural identity to embrace the international medical conference style. This standardization is part of the globalization that we are all witnessing.

The most widely spoken language is not Chinese, English or Spanish anymore, but the new phenomenon of broken English. This language is the result of simplifying English to make it as neutral and understandable as possible, removing colloquial idioms, regional expressions or any other source of linguistic confusion.

In this new universe, health-care professionals find themselves having to make a conscious effort to adapt to these explicit and implicit rules. Some of them are discussed in the following sections.

Having read this chapter you will not only be able to improve your presentations or feel at ease giving them, but you might also actually end up being able to convey your message and, who knows? ... you might even enjoy it – even if you have to deliver your presentation in the graveyard slot (the graveyard slot is the first presentation after lunch when most of the audience will be suffering from postprandial somnolence and very likely you will not hear a sound except for snores).

Dos and Don'ts

Time is also a very cultural thing. This peculiarity should be taken into account. Eight o'clock in the morning might seem an early start in Latin America but a perfectly normal starting time in northern Europe and the US. Furthermore, the day is divided differently in various parts of the world ... and in our radiological universe. Thus at an international conference the day is divided into:

- The morning: from the start time to noon.
- The afternoon: from 12:01 to 17:00 or 18:00.
- The evening: from 18:00 to midnight.

- *Do* remember to follow these tips:
  - *Good morning*: from the start time to 12:00.
  - *Good afternoon*: from 12:01 onwards, even though your metabolism is far from feeling afternoon-ish until your usual lunch time has gone by and is begging you to say "good morning".
  - *Good evening*: from 18:00 onwards. Note that if we have to give a presentation, make a speech or offer a toast at 22:00, we should never begin with "good night"; that should be reserved only for when we are going to bed. So "good night" is not supposed to be said in public.

When giving a presentation, there is always a time limit. I understand, and have actually experienced myself, how difficult it is to cram all we have to say about the topic which we have been researching over the last few years into a mere 20 minutes. In view of this time constraint, there are various alternatives ranging from speaking as fast as the tongue can rattle, to cutting it down to 5 minutes and spending the other 15 minutes vacantly gazing at the audience. American, British and Australian physicians are often extremely fluent speakers (we know, we know ... they are using their mother tongue). However, remember that showing and commenting on five slides a minute and speaking faster than can be registered on a digital recorder might not be the best way of conveying a message.

- *Don't* speak too fast or too slowly.
- *Don't* say sorry for this slide. Since you are the one who chooses the slides to be presented, get rid of those you would have to apologize for.
- *Do* summarize your presentation and rehearse to see how long you need for a clear delivery.

Sometimes lecturers tend to give too much data and minor details in their presentations. Their introduction is often full of information that is of little relevance to the international audience (for example, the name, date and code of local, provincial, regional and national laws regulating radiological standards in his/her institution; or even the background information on the main researchers of a trial including their graduation year and shoe size ... or a full history of the 16th Century building where the hospital stands today and subsequent restorations it has undergone; etc). In these cases, by the time all these details have been given and the presentation has passed the introduction stage, time is up and the chairperson starts making desperate signs to the speaker.

- *Do* grab the pointer with both hands.

The best way of avoiding a trembling pointer is to grab it with both hands and place them over the lectern. If this doesn't work, we recommend using the mouse since, at least, your trembling will be confined to one plane instead of the three-dimensional shaking of a laser pointer.

- *Do* use either a pointer or the computer's mouse.

Although it may seem unbelievable, I attended a lecture in which the presenter instead of using a laser pointer directed the audience's attention to the images using a folded newspaper. The only person who could see the details the speaker was pointing out was the speaker himself.

- *Do* structure your presentation so that you convey a few clear messages instead of a huge amount of not-so-relevant information which nobody has a chance to take in.
- *Don't* read slides, but instead try to explain a few basic ideas as clearly as possible.

Many intermediate English-speaking doctors could not agree with this point because they can only feel some confidence if they read the presentation. Reading is the least-natural means of communicating experiences; we encourage you to present your paper without reading it. Although it will need much more intensive preparation, the delivery will be more fluid and – why not? – even brilliant. Many foreign doctors resign themselves to delivering just acceptable talks and explicitly reject the possibility of making a presentation at the same level as they would in their own language. Do not reject the possibility of being as brilliant as you would be in your own language; the only difference is in the amount of rehearsal. Thorough rehearsal can provide you with amazing results; do not give up beforehand.

- *Don't* read your presentation from a script.

Even worse than reading slides is to read from a script. I have witnessed complete messes happening to lecturers who tried, without any success at all, to coordinate scribbled pages on the lectern and slides. The noise of the passing pages was unbearable and the face of a speaker on the verge of a mental breakdown kept the audience from listening to the presentation itself.

- *Do* enjoy yourself.

When giving the presentation, relax; nobody knows more than you do about the specific subject that you are presenting. The only way to make people enjoy your presentation is by enjoying it yourself. You only have to communicate, not to perform; being a good researcher or a competent clinician is not the same thing as being a stand-up comedian or a model. This does not mean that we can afford to overlook our presentation skills, especially if you want most of your colleagues to still be awake at the end of your presentation!

- *Do* try to overcome stage fright and focus on communicating.

There must be somebody out there interested in what you have to say ... either to praise it or to tear it to pieces, but that doesn't matter.

- *Do* avoid anything that would make you nervous when giving your presentation.

One piece of advice is to remove all keys, coins or other metal objects from your pockets so that you are not tempted to rattle them around – a truly irritating noise that we have all learned to hate.

- *Do* put your cell phone (*UK* mobile phone) and beeper on silent.

The only thing more embarrassing than an attendee's cell phone interrupting your lecture is your own phone ringing in the middle of your talk.

- *Do* make sure that your jokes can be understood internationally.

Creativity and humor are always appreciated in a lecture hall ... providing they are both appropriate and understood! We all know that humor is a very cultural thing, like time keeping, ties, food preferences, etc. Almost all American speakers will start their presentation with a joke that most Europeans will not understand, not even the Irish or British. A British speaker will probably throw in the most sarcastic comment when you are least expecting it and in the same tone as if he or she were telling you about the mortality rate in his or her unit. A foreign (neither American nor British) doctor might just try to tell a long joke in English based on a play on words in his or her mother tongue which obviously doesn't work in English, and possibly involves religion, sport and/or sex (as a general rule avoid religious and sex jokes in public presentations).

Useful Sentences for Radiological Talks

Introducing the Presentation

- Good afternoon. It is an honor to have the opportunity to speak to you about ...
- Good afternoon. Thank you for your kind introduction. It is my pleasure to speak to you about an area of great interest to me.
- In the next few minutes I'll talk about ...
- The topic I'll cover this afternoon is ...
- In the next 20 minutes I'll show you ...
- In my talk on focal hepatic lesions, I want to share with you all our experience on ...
- Thank you for sticking around (informal way of addressing the last talk attendees).

- I'd like to thank you Dr. Ho for his kind invitation.
- Thank you Dr. Wilson for inviting me to attend this course.
- Thank you Dr. Olsen. It is a great honor to be here talking about …
- On behalf of my colleagues and assistants, I want to thank Dr. Smith for his kind invitation.
- I'd like to welcome you to this course on … (to be said in the first talk of the course if you are a member of the organizing committee)
- Today, I want to talk to you about …
- Now, allow me to introduce …
- What I want to talk about this morning is …
- During the next few minutes, I'd like to draw your attention to …
- First of all, let me summarize the contents of my lecture on …
- Let's begin by looking at these 3D images of the heart …

Commenting on Images, Graphs, Tables, Schematic Representations …

- As you can see in the image on your right …
- As you will see in the next table …
- As we saw in the previous slide …
- The next image shows …
- The next image allows us to …
- In the bottom left image we can see …
- What do we have to look at here?
- What do we have to bear in mind with regard to this artifact?
- Notice how the lesion borders are …
- Bear in mind that this image was obtained in less than 10 seconds …
- Let's look at this schematic representation of the portal vein …
- As you can see in this CT image …
- Let us have a look at this schematic diagram of the portal system …
- Looking at this table, you can see …
- Having a look at this bar chart, we could conclude that …
- To sum up, let's look at this diagram …
- The image on your right …
- The image at the top of the screen shows …
- Let's turn to the next slide in which the lesion, after the administration of contrast material, is more conspicuous …
- Figure 7 brings out the importance of …
- As can be observed in this MR image …
- I apologize that the faint area of sclerosis in the femur *does not project well*. (When a subtle finding is difficult to see on a projected image, it is said that *it does not project well*.)

- On the left of the screen is a T2-weighted image at the level of the pons. On the right of the screen there is a *magnified view* of the abnormality.

Summing Up

- To sum up we can say that ...
- In summary, we have discussed ...
- To conclude ...
- Summing up, I would say that ...
- The take-home lesson of the talk is ...
- To put it in a nutshell ...
- To cut a long story short ...
- In short, ...
- To put it briefly ...
- Be that as it may, we have to bear in mind that ...
- If there is one point I hope you will take away from this presentation, it is that ...
- CT has proven to be very useful in the assessment of lung cancer by providing additional information during image interpretation.
- Cardiac CT is a powerful technique that yields valuable diagnostic information.
- The rate of growth and distribution of cardiac CT will depend on investing in technology, training, and collaboration.
- MRI may be helpful in the management of ... if sonography is inconclusive.
- Virtual colonoscopy is the most accurate technique for the assessment of ...

Concluding

- Thank you for your kind attention.
- Thank you all for sticking around until the very last talk of the session.
- Thank you all.
- Thank you very much for your time, you have been a most gracious audience.
- Thank you for your attention. I would be happy to entertain any questions.
- Thank you for your time. I would be happy to address any questions.

- This is all we have time for, so thank you and have a good time in London.
- Let me finish my presentation by saying that …
- We can say to conclude that …
- Let me end by wishing you a pleasant stay in our city.
- I'd be happy to answer any question you might have.
- I'd be happy to address your comments and questions.
- Ignore lesions less than 4 mm in your reports.

The Dreadful Questions and Comments Section

Many beginners would not hesitate to deliver a free communication at an international congress if there were not a short section of questions after them.

This anecdote may illustrate the feelings of many non-native English-speaking radiologists in their first presentations in English.

After a short free communication on the MR follow-up of Ross operation (the surgical replacement of a patient's aortic valve by the pulmonary valve and the replacement of the latter by a homograft) which had so far gone reasonably well for a beginner, I was waiting, like a rabbit staring at a snake, for the round of questions that inevitably followed my presentation.

On the very verge of a mental breakdown, I listened to an English radiologist asking me a question I could barely understand. I told him: "would you please repeat your question?", and he, obediently, repeated the question with exactly the same words and the same pace with which he had formulated it before. As I could not understand the question the second time, the chairman roughly translated it into a more international and easily understandable English and I finally answered it. This was the only question I was asked since the time was over and there was no room for any other comment.

Let us think about this anecdote in a positive way by dissecting it into the following points which will lead us to some recommendations.

1. Do not be discouraged. Nobody told you that beginnings were easy.
2. Questions and comments by native English speakers tend to be more difficult to understand.
3. There are several types of interlocutors you must be aware of.
4. Do not complain if the interlocutor does exactly what you asked him/her for.
5. Chairmen can always help you.
6. Time is limited and you can take advantage of this fact.

These points lead to some recommendations:
1. I did not know by then that the worst was still to come. I wasted the whole morning recreating the scene over and over. "How could I have spoiled so many hours of research and study? I even thought that people recognized me as "the one who didn't understand a simple query ..."

   Let us think for a moment how you performed the first time you did anything in your life, i.e., the first time you grabbed a tennis racquet or a golf club. In comparison to that it was not that bad.

2. When the radiologist who asked for the microphone is a non-native English speaker you can begin to feel better since you are going to talk to an equal with regard to language, to one who has spent a great number of hours fighting to learn a language other than his own. On the other hand, when you have to deal with a native English speaker there are two main types of interlocutors.

   Type A is a colleague who does not take advantage of being a native English speaker and reduces his normal rhythm of speech so you can understand the question and, therefore, convey to the audience whatever you have to say.

   Type B is a colleague who does not make any allowance for the difference between native and non-native English lecturers. Needless to say, I faced a type B interlocutor in my first international presentation.

3. Types of interlocutors:
   - *Type 1*: The interlocutor who wants to know a particular detail of your presentation. These interlocutors are easy to handle by just answering their questions.

     What diameters do you measure in the aortic root?
     Annulus, Valsalva sinuses, and sinotubular junction.

   - *Type 2*: The interlocutor who wants the audience to notice his sound knowledge of the subject which is being discussed. These interlocutors are quite easy to handle as well since they do not formulate questions as such but make a point of their own. The replies tend to be shorter than the questions/comments and time, which runs in favor of the beginner provided he is not speaking, goes by, leaving no room for another dreadful question.

     I do agree with your comments
     We are planning to include this point in our next paper on ...

   - *Type 3*: The interlocutor who strongly disagrees with your points. This is obviously the most difficult to handle for a beginner due to the scarcity of his idiomatic resources. The only piece of advice is none other than that you must defend your points from a humble position and do not ever challenge your interlocutor.

I will consider your suggestions on ...
This is a work in progress and we will consider including your suggestions ...

4. If I had requested my interlocutor to ask his question again more slowly and in a different way so I could understand it he would have been morally obliged to do so. But beginners lack this kind of modesty and pretend to be better and know more than they actually are and do, which is, by definition, a mistake.

I don't understand your question. Would you please reformulate your question in a different way, please?

5. When you feel you need some help, ask the chairman to help you out.

Dr. Ho (chairman) I'm not sure I've understood the question. Would you please formulate it in a different way?

6. It is, at worst, 1 minute of stress. Do not let such a short period of time prevent you from a potentially successful career in international radiology.

Sentences That May Help

Go over these sentences that may help you escape from a difficult situation and minimize your fear of the questions and comments section:

Making Your Point

- Let me point out that signal intensity is paramount in order to differentiate ...
- You must bear in mind that this 3D reconstruction was obtained ...
- If you look closely at this brain tumor, you will realize that ...
- I want to draw your attention to the fact that ...
- Don't forget the importance of SPIO in ...
- Before I move on to my next slide ...
- In view of the upcoming publication of ...
- Radiologically speaking ...
- From a radiological point of view ...
- As far as trackability is concerned ...
- The bottom line of the subject is ...

Giving Explanations

- To put it another way, chemical shift artifact was responsible for ...
- Taking into consideration that the study was done under conscious sedation ...
- In a bit more detail, you can notice that ...
- This fact can be explained taking into account that ...
- SNR (signal-to-noise ratio) was poor since the patient could not hold his breath.
- Although double phospho-soda was well tolerated by most patients ...
- In short, you may need larger balloons in elderly patients.
- What I'm saying is that endometriosis is related to ectopic growth of endometrial tissue ...
- We did not administer contrast material because the patient refused it.
- We perform an unenhanced CT scan because the patient suffered from renal insufficiency.

Answering Multiple Questions

- There are two different questions here.
- It seems there are three questions here.
- It is my understanding that there are two questions to be addressed here.
- With regard to your first question ...
- Regarding your second question ...
- As far as your first question is concerned ...
- Answering your first question, I should say that ...
- I'll begin with your second question.
- Let me address your last question first.
- I'll address your last question first and then the rest of them.
- Would you please repeat your second question?
- I didn't understand your first question. Would you repeat it?

Disagreeing

- With all due respect, I believe that there is no evidence of ...
- To the best of our knowledge no article has been published on this topic.
- With all respect, I think that your point overlooks the main aspect of ...
- Yours is an interesting point of view, but I'm not sure of its ...

- I see it from a different point of view.
- With all respect, I don't go along with you on ...
- I think that the importance of ... cannot be denied.
- I strongly disagree with your comment on ...
- I disagree with your point.
- I don't see a valid argument for supporting such a comment.

Emphasizing a Point

- I do believe that ...
- I strongly agree with Dr. Ho's comments on ...
- It is of paramount importance ...
- It is a crucial fact that ...
- And this fact cannot be overlooked.
- I'd like to stress the importance of ...
- Don't underestimate the role of ...
- The use of iodinated contrast material in these cases is of the utmost importance.
- With regard to ..., you must always bear in mind that ...
- It is well known that ...

Incomprehension

- I'm not sure I understood your question ...
- Sorry; I don't quite follow you.
- Would you repeat the question, please?
- Would you repeat the second part of your question, please?
- I'm afraid I still don't understand.
- Could you be a bit more specific with regard to ...?
- What do you mean by ...?
- Could you repeat your question? I couldn't hear you.
- Could you formulate your question in a different way?
- I'm not sure I understand your final question.

Playing for Time

- I am not sure I understood your question. Would you repeat it?
- I don't understand your questions. Would you formulate it in a different way?
- That's a very interesting question ...
- I wonder if you could be a bit more specific about ...

- I'm glad you asked that question.
- Your question is of the utmost importance, but I'm afraid it is beyond the scope of our paper ...
- What aspect of the problem are you referring to by saying ...

Evading an Issue

- I'm afraid I'm not really in a position to be able to address your question yet.
- We'll come back to that in a minute, if you don't mind.
- I don't think we have enough time to discuss your comments in depth.
- It would take extremely long time to answer that.
- I will address your question in my second talk, if you don't mind.
- At my institution, we do not have experience on ...
- At our department, we do not perform ...
- Perhaps we could return to that at the end of the session.
- We'll probably address your question in further papers on the subject.
- I have no experience ...

Technical Problems

- May I have another laser pointer?
- Does anyone in the audience have a pointer?
- Video images are not running properly. In the meantime I'd like to comment on ...
- My microphone is not working properly. May I have it fixed?
- My microphone is not working properly. May I use yours?
- Can you hear me?
- Can the rows at the back hear me?
- Can you guys at the back see the screen?
- Can we turn off the lights please?

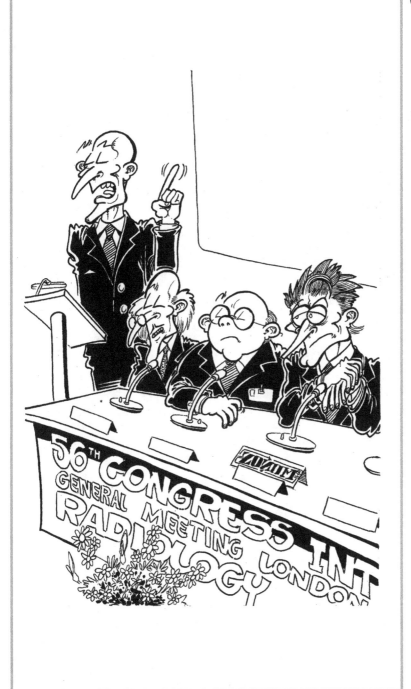

Unit VII   Chairing a Radiological Session

Chairing sessions at international meetings usually comes up when you have reached a certain level in your academic career. To reach this point many papers will have been submitted and many presentations will have been given, so the chances are your level of medical English will be above that of the target audience of this manual.

Why, then, do we include a section on chairing a session?

We include it because contrary to what many of those who have never chaired a session in an international meeting may think, even an experienced chairperson may face difficult, even embarrassing situations.

For those who have never chaired a session, to be a chairman means, firstly, not having to prepare a presentation, and, secondly, the use of simple sentences such as "thank you, Dr. Vida, for your interesting presentation" or "the next speaker will be Dr. Jones who comes from ...".

In our opinion, being a chairperson means much more than one who has never chaired them might think. To begin with, a chairperson must go over not one presentation but thoroughly study all the recently published material on the subject under discussion. On top of that, a chairperson must review all the abstracts and must have prepared questions just in case the audience has no questions or comments.

We have divided this section into four subsections:

1. Usual chairperson's comments.
2. Should chairpersons ask questions?
3. What the chairperson should say when something is going wrong.
4. Specific radiological chairperson's comments

Usual Chairperson's Comments

Everybody who has attended an international meeting is aware of the usual sentences the chairperson uses to introduce the session. Certain key expressions will provide you with a sense of fluency without which chairing a session would be troublesome. The good news is that if you know the key sentences and use them appropriately, chairing a session is easy. The bad news is that if, on the contrary, you do not know these expressions, a theoretically simple task will become an embarrassing situation. There is always a first time for everything, and if it is the first time you have been invited to chair a session, rehearse some of these sentences and you will feel quite comfortable. Accept this piece of advice: only "rehearsed spontaneity" looks spontaneous if you are a beginner.

Introducing the Session

We suggest the following useful comments for introducing the session:

- Good morning ladies and gentlemen. My name is Dr. Vida and I want to welcome you all to this workshop on congenital heart disease imaging. My co-chair is Dr. Vick who comes from King's College.
- Good afternoon. The session on MRI in cardiomyopathies is about to start. Please take a seat and disconnect your cellular phones and any other electrical devices which could interfere with the oral presentations. We will listen to ten six-minute lectures with a two-minute period for questions and comments after each, and afterwards, provided we are still on time, we will have a last round of questions and comments from the audience, speakers and panelists.
- Good morning. We will proceed with the session on fibroid embolization. As many papers have to be delivered I encourage the speakers to keep an eye on the time.

Introducing Speakers

We suggest the following useful comments for introducing speakers:

- Our first speaker is Dr. Vida from Reina Sofia Hospital in Cordoba, Spain, who will present the paper: "MR evaluation of focal splenic lesions".

The following speakers are introduced almost the same way with sentences such as:

- Our next lecturer is Dr. Adams. Dr. Adams comes from Brigham and Women's Hospital. Harvard Medical School, and his presentation is entitled "Diagnosis of intraosseous ganglion".
- Next is Dr. Shaw from Beth Israel Deaconess Hospital, presenting "MR approaches to molecular imaging".
- Dr. Olsen from UCSF is the next and last speaker. His presentation is: "Metastatic disease. Pathways to the heart".

Once the speakers finish their presentation, the chairperson is supposed to say something like:

- Thank you Dr. Vida for your excellent presentation. Any questions or comments?

The chairperson usually comments on presentations, although sometimes they do not:

- Thank you Dr. Vida for your presentation. Are there any questions or comments from the audience?

There are some common adjectives (*nice, elegant, outstanding, excellent, interesting, clear, accurate* ...) and formulas that are usually used to describe presentations. These are illustrated in the following comments:

- Thanks Dr. Shaw for your accurate presentation. Does the audience have any comments?
- Thank you very much for your clear presentation on this always controversial topic. I would like to ask a question. May I? (Although being the chairperson you are the one who gives permission, to ask the speaker is a usual formality.)
- I'd like to thank you for this excellent talk Dr. Olsen. Any questions?
- Thanks a lot for your talk Dr. Ho. I wonder if the audience has got any questions?

Adjourning

We suggest the following useful comments for adjourning the session:

- I think we all are a bit tired so we'll have a short break.
- The session is adjourned until 4 p.m.
- We'll take a short break.
- We'll take a 30-minute break. Please fill out the evaluation forms.
- The session is adjourned until tomorrow morning. Enjoy your stay in Vienna.

Finishing the Session

We suggest the following useful comments for finishing the session:

- I'd like to thank all the speakers and the audience for your interesting presentations and comments. (I'll) see you all at the congress dinner and awards ceremony.
- The session is over. I want to thank all the participants for their contribution. (I'll) see you tomorrow morning. Remember to take your attendance certificates if you have not taken them already.
- We should finish up over here. We'll resume at 10:50.

Should Chairpersons Ask Questions?

In our opinion, chairpersons are supposed to ask questions especially at the beginning of the session when the audience does not usually make any comments at all. Warming-up the session is one of the chairperson's duties, and if nobody in the audience is in the mood to ask questions the chairperson must invite the audience to participate:

* Are there any questions?

Nobody raises their hand:

* Well, I have got two questions for Dr. Adams. Do you think MR is the imaging method of choice for the detection and characterization of focal splenic lesions? and second: What should be, in your opinion, the role of CT and ultrasound in this diagnostic algorithm?

Once the session has been warmed-up, the chairperson should only ask questions or add comments as a tool to manage the timing of the session, so that, if as usual, the session is behind schedule, the chairperson is not required to participate unless strictly necessary.

The chairperson does not have to demonstrate to the audience his or her knowledge on the discussed topics by asking too many questions or making comments. The chairperson's knowledge of the subject is not in doubt since without it he or she would not have been selected to chair.

What the Chairperson Should Say when Something is Going Wrong

Behind Schedule

Many lecturers, knowing beforehand they have a certain amount of time to deliver their presentations, try to talk a little bit more, stealing time from the questions/comments time and from later speakers. Chairpersons should cut short this tendency at the very first chance:

* Dr. Berlusconi, your time is almost over. You have got 30 seconds to finish your presentation.
* Dr. Ho, you are running out of time.

If the speaker does not finish his presentation on time, the chairperson may say:

* Dr. Berlusconi, I'm sorry but your time is over. We must proceed to the next presentation. Any questions, comments?

After introducing the next speaker, sentences such as the following will help you handle the session:

- Dr. Goyen, please keep an eye on the time, we are behind schedule.
- We are far from being ahead of schedule, so I remind all speakers you have six minutes to deliver your presentation.

Ahead of Schedule

Although unusual, sometimes there is some extra time and this is a good chance to ask the panelists a general question about their experience at their respective institutions:

- As we are a little bit ahead of schedule, I encourage the panelists and the audience to ask questions and offer comments.
- I have got a question for the panelists: What percentage of the total number of CMRs at your institution are performed on children?

Technical Problems

Computer Not Working

We suggest the following comments:

- I am afraid there is a technical problem with the computer. In the meantime I would like to make a comment about ...
- The computer is not working properly. While it is being fixed I encourage the panelists to offer their always interesting comments.

Lights Gone Out

We suggest the following comments:

- The lights have gone out. We'll take a hopefully short break until they are repaired.
- As you see, or indeed do not see at all, the lights have gone out. The hotel staff have told us it is going to be a matter of minutes so do not go too far; we'll resume as soon as possible.

Sound Gone Off

We suggest the following comments:

- Dr. Hoffman, we cannot hear you. There must be a problem with your microphone.
- Perhaps you could try this microphone?
- Please would you use the microphone, the rows at the back cannot hear you.

Lecturer Lacks Confidence

If the lecturer is speaking too quietly:

- Dr. Smith would you please speak up? The audience cannot hear you.
- Dr. Alvarez would you please speak up a bit? The people at the back cannot hear you.

If the lecturer is so nervous he/she cannot go on delivering the presentation:

- Dr. Olsen, take your time. We can proceed to the next presentation, so whenever you feel OK and ready to deliver yours, it will be a pleasure to listen to it.

Specific Radiological Chairperson's Comments

Since chairpersons are supposed to fill in the gaps in the session, if a technical problem occurs, the chairperson must say something "to entertain" the audience in the meantime. This fact would not create any problem to a native English speaker but may be troublesome for a non-native English-speaking chairperson. In these situations there is an always helpful topic to be addressed "in the meantime", namely, the current situation of what is discussed in the session in the panelists' countries.

- Regarding CMR, how are things going in Italy, Dr. Toldo?
- As for as the use of SPIO, what's the deal in Japan, Dr. Hashimoto?
- How is the current situation in Germany regarding repayment policies?
- May I ask how many CMR studies you are performing yearly at your respective institutions?
- What's going on in the States, Dr. Olsen?

By opening a discussion on how things are going in different countries, the not-too-fluent chairperson shares the burden of filling in the gaps with the panelists. This trick rarely fails and once the technical problem is fixed the session can go on normally with nobody in the audience noticing the lack of fluency of the chairperson.

Besides the usual expressions chairpersons of whatever medical specialty have to be aware of, there are typical comments a radiological chairperson should be familiar with. These comments vary depending upon the radiological subspecialty of the chairperson and are, generally speaking, easy to deal with for even non-native English speakers. By way of example, let's review the following:

- Dr. Petit, would you please use the pointer so the audience know what lesion you are talking about?

- Dr. Wilson, would you please point out the borders of the lesion so we can distinguish the tumor from the surrounding edema?
- Dr. Negroponte, did you perform an abdominal ultrasound scan on this patient?
- Dr. Maier, did you perform the brain MR on an emergent basis?
- Have you had any adverse anaphylactic reactions to this type of contrast material?
- Dr. Olsen, I can't see the lesion you are talking about. Can you point it out?
- Do you use 12F catheters for this purpose?
- Dr. Pons, I'm afraid that the video is not running properly. Could you try to fix it so we can see your excellent cardiac MR images?
- Dr. Hashimoto, why didn't you use a 0.0035 stiff guidewire to cross the stenosis?
- Dr. Soares, are you currently using gadolinium in cases like this one?
- Dr. Mas, is trackability that important in these cases?
- Do you do enhanced lumbosacral spine MRs in all postoperative patients?
- Do you perform preprocedure pelvic MRI in all patients undergoing uterine artery embolization?

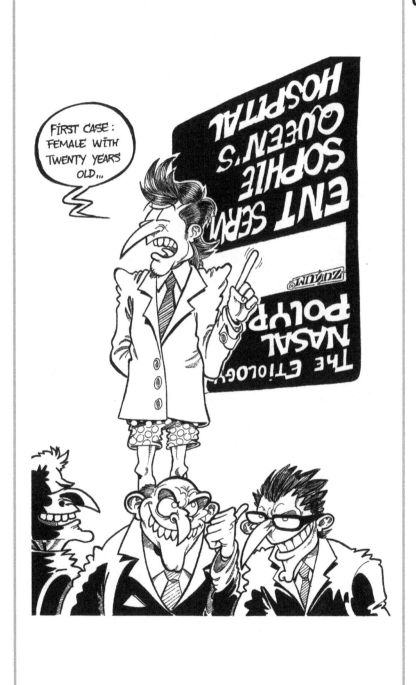

Unit VIII   Usual Mistakes Made by Radiologists Speaking and Writing in English

In this section we try to share with you what we have found to be some of the great hurdles in radiological English. There are many things that certainly can go wrong when one is asked to give a lecture in English or whenever one is supposed to communicate in radiological English. This is by no means an exhaustive account, it is just a way of passing on what we have learnt from our own experience in the fascinating world of radiological English.

When preparing and actually delivering a presentation in English at an international radiological conference, a series of basic issues should be taken into account. We have grouped them into four danger zones, in the hope that their classification will make them become less of a problem. The categories are the following:

1. Misnomers and false friends
2. Common grammatical mistakes
3. Common spelling mistakes
4. Common pronunciation mistakes.

Misnomers and False Friends

Every tongue has its own false friends. A thorough review of false friends is beyond the scope of this manual, and we suggest that you look for those tricky names that sound similar in your language and in English but have completely different meanings.

Think, for example, about the term *graft versus host disease*. The translation of *host* has not been correct in some romance languages, and in Spanish the term *host*, which in this context means recipient, has been translated as *huésped* which means *person staying in another's house*. Many Spanish medical students have problems with the understanding of this disease because of the terminology used. Taking into account that what actually happens is that the graft reacts against the recipient, if the disease had been named *graft versus recipient disease*, the concept would probably be more precisely conveyed.

So from now on, identify false friends in your own language and make a list beginning with those belonging to your specialty; it is no use knowing false friends in a language different from your own.

Medicine, in general, and anatomy and radiology in particular, are full of misnomers. Think for a moment about the term *superficial femoral vein*. It is difficult to explain how a superficial femoral vein clot is actually in the deep venous system.

Many radiologists and oncologists all over the world say *small (mediastinal) lymphadenopathies*. Taking into account that size is the only criterion for the diagnosis of abnormal lymph nodes (the usefulness of USPIO in the diagnosis of lymphadenopathies is beyond the scope of this manual) and that lymphadenopathy means, from an etymological point of view, abnormal lymph node, a *"normal" (small size) lymphadenopathy* is as absurd as a *normal psychopathy*. The term *lymphadenomegaly* would probably be a more accurate one.

Etymologically *pancreas* means *all meat*, but there is no muscle at all in that endocrine and exocrine gland.

Why do we call the innermost part of the elbow which is medial and slightly proximal to the trochlea the *medial epicondyle* instead of *epitrochlea*?

Etymologically *azygos* means *odd* which puts *hemiazygos* in a strange situation since odd numbers are not divisible by two.

The term *innominate vein* is as absurd as naming a baby *unnamed*.

Common Grammatical Mistakes

These are some of the most common mistakes made by radiologists speaking in English:

1. The axial fast spin echo T2 image through the patella showed an enlarged and thickened medial patellar plica.
   MR images have by definition T1, PD, and T2 information so, after the predominant weighting, the use of "-weighted image" is imperative. The correct sentence would be:
   • The axial fast spin echo T2-weighted image through the patella showed an enlarged and thickened medial patellar plica.

2. The intact posterior cruciate ligament was isointense and presented no signs of disruption.
   Isointensity is always a relative magnitude so the correct sentence in this case would be:
   • The intact posterior cruciate ligament was isointense to cortical bone and showed no signs of disruption.

3. The cyst was hyperintense in T2-weighted images.
   Although you may have seen this expression in some talks, it is more correct to say:
   • The cyst was hyperintense on T2-weighted images.

4. A MR magnet was purchased by the hospital.
   Although *a magnetic resonance magnet* ... is correct, when you use the acronym do not forget that "m" is read "em" which starts with a vowel, so the article to be used is "an" instead of "a". In this case you should write:
   * An MR magnet was purchased by the hospital.

5. The chairman of radiology came from an university hospital.
   Although university starts with a vowel, and you may think the article which must precede it is "an" as in "an airport", the "u" is pronounced "you" which starts with a consonant, so the article to be used is "a" instead of "an". In this case you should write:
   * The chairman of radiology came from a university hospital.

6. A 22-years-old man presenting ...
   Many times the first sentence of the first slide of a presentation contains the first error. For those lecturers at an intermediate level, this simple mistake is so evident that they barely believe it is one of the most frequent mistakes ever made.
   It is quite obvious that the adjective *22-year-old* cannot be written in the plural and it should be written:
   * A 22-year-old man presenting ...

7. There was not biopsy of the lesion.
   This is a frequent and relatively subtle mistake made by upper-intermediate speakers. If you still prefer the use of the negative form you should say:
   * There was not *any* biopsy of the lesion.
   But the affirmative form is:
   * There was no biopsy of the lesion.

8. It allows to distinguish between ...
   You should use one of the following phrases:
   * It allows us to distinguish between ...
   or
   * It allows the distinction between ...

9. Haemorrhagic tumors can cause.
   Check your paper or presentation for inconsistency in the use of American and British English.
   This example shows a sentence made up of an American English word (*tumors*) and a British English word (*haemorrhagic*). So choose American or British spelling depending on the journal or congress you are sending your paper to.
   The sentence should read:
   * Haemorrhagic tumours can cause.
   or
   * Hemorrhagic tumors can cause.

10. Please would you tell me where is the IR suite?

   Embedded questions are always troublesome. Whenever a question is embedded in another interrogative sentence its word order changes. This happens when, trying to be polite, we incorrectly change *What time is it?* to *Would you please tell me what time is it?* instead of to *Would you please tell me what time it is?*

   The direct question *where is the IR suite?* must be transformed to its embedded form as follows:

   • Please would you tell me where the IR suite is?

11. Most of the times hemangiomas ...

   You can say *many times* but not *most of the times. Most of the time* is correct and you can use *commonly* or *frequently* as equivalent terms. Say instead:

   • Most of the time hemangiomas ...

12. I look forward to hear from you.

   This a very frequent mistake at the end of formal letters such as those sent to editors. The mistake is based upon a grammatical error. *To* may be either a part of the infinitive or a preposition. In this case *to* is not a part of the infinitive of the verb *hear* but a part of the prepositional verb *look forward to*; it is indeed a preposition.

   There may be irreparable consequences of making this mistake. If you are trying to have an article published in a prestigious journal you cannot make formal mistakes which can preclude the reading of your otherwise interesting article.

   So instead of *look forward to hear from you*, you should write:

   • I look forward to hearing from you.

13. Best regards.

   Although it is used in both academic and informal correspondence *best regards* is a mixture of two strong English collocations: *kind regards* and *best wishes*. In our opinion instead of *best regards*, which is colloquially acceptable, you should write:

   • Kind regards

   or simply

   • Regards.

14. Are you suffering from paresthesias?

   Many doctors forget that patients are not colleagues and use medical terminology which cannot be understood by them. This technical question would be easily understood in the form:

   • Do you have pins and needles?

15. A unique metastases was seen in the liver.

   Unique and metastases are incompatible terms since the former refers to singular and the latter to plural. Therefore, the appropriate sentence should have been:

   • A unique metastasis was seen in the liver.

16. Multiple metastasis were seen in the brain.

Multiple and metastases are incompatible terms since the former refers to plural and the latter to singular. Whenever you use a Latin term check its singular and plural. Metastasis is singular whereas metastases is plural so that *there are multiple metastasis* is not correct. In this case, you should write:

- Multiple metastases were seen in the brain.

17. An European expert on cardiac MR chaired the session.

Although European starts with a vowel and you may think the article which must precede it is "an" as in "an airport", the correct sentence, in this case, would be:

- A European expert on cardiac MR chaired the session.

18. The meeting began a hour ago.

Although hour starts with a consonant and you may think the article which must precede it is "a" as in "a cradle", the correct sentence, in this case, would be:

- The meeting began an hour ago.

Words starting with a silent "h" are preceded by "an" as if they started with a vowel.

19. The cardiac surgeon who asked for the CMR was operating the stenotic aortic valve reported as such by the radiologist.

This sentence is not correct since the verb "to operate" when is used from a surgical point of view (with regard to both patients and parts of the anatomy) is always followed by the preposition "on". The correct sentence would have been:

- The cardiac surgeon who asked for the CMR was operating on the stenotic aortic valve reported as such by the radiologist.

20. Medial and collateral ligaments are well defined on the coronal plane.

We use "in" when talking about planes (coronal, axial, sagittal …) since the radiological finding is within the image. So, although acceptable, it would have been better to say:

- Medial and collateral ligaments are well defined in the coronal plane.

21. The hospital personal are very kind.

When we talk about a group of people working at an institution, the correct word is "personnel", not "personal":

- The hospital personnel are very kind.

22. Page to the cardiologist.

The verb "to page" which could be related to the substantive "page" (a boy who is employed to run errands) is not a prepositional verb and does not need the preposition "to" after it. When you want the cardiologist paged you must say:

- Page the cardiologist.

23. She works in the neurorradiology division.
    This is a common mistake made by Spanish and Latin American radiologists. In English, neuroradiology is written with one "r":
    • She works in the neuroradiology division.

Common Spelling Mistakes

Create your own list of potentially misspelled words and don't hesitate to write down you own mnemonic if it helps you.

The following is a list of commonly misspelled words (with the most common misspelling given in parentheses):

• Parallel (misspelled: paralell)

For this frequently misspelled word, I use this quite absurd (as most mnemonics are) mnemonic to recall the spelling: "two Legs (ll) run faster, and get forward, than one (l)".

• Appearance (misspelled: apperance)

We've seen this mistake more than once in radiological drafts. The only thing you have to check to avoid it is that the verb "appear" is embedded in the word "appearance"

• Sagittal (misspelled: saggital)

In a word with double consonants and single consonants, avoid doubling the single consonant and vice versa. Sagittal is one of the most commonly misspelled words in radiological slides. Words such as sagittal are among the most frequently used in radiology. The etymology of this word is *sagita* which means "arrow".

• Dura mater (misspelled: dura matter)

Etymologically "mater" means "mother" and is written with one "t". "Dura matter" is a common mistake based upon the mixing up of "dura mater" and "gray/white matter". "Matter" means substance and has nothing to do with "mater".

• Arrhythmia (misspelled: arrhytmia)

Double-check the spelling of arrhythmia and be sure that the word "rhythm" from which it is derived is embedded in it.
    Review the following further pairs of words (with the misspelling given in parentheses) and, more importantly, as we said above, create your own list of "troublesome" words.

- Professor (misspelled: proffesor)
- Professional (misspelled: proffesional)
- Occasion (misspelled: ocassion)
- Dissection (misspelled: disection)
- Resection (misspelled: ressection)
- Gray-white matter (misspelled: gray-white mater)
- Subtraction (misspelled: substraction)
- Acquisition (misspelled: adquisition)

Common Pronunciation Mistakes

For simplicity, we have taken the liberty of using an approximate representation of the pronunciation instead of using the phonetic signs. We apologize to our linguist colleagues who may have preferred a more orthodox transcription.

Pronunciation is one of the most dreaded nightmares of English. Although there are pronunciation rules, there are so many exceptions that you must know the pronunciation of most words by ear. Therefore, firstly, read out loud as much as you can because it is the only way you will notice the unknown words with regard to pronunciation, and secondly, when you attend a course, besides concentrating on the presentation itself, focus on the way native-English-speaking radiologists pronounce the words you do not know.

With regard to pronunciation, we recommend that you should:

- Not be afraid of sounding different or funny. English sounds *are* different and funny. Sometimes a non-native-speaking radiologist may know how to pronounce a word correctly but is a bit ashamed of doing so, particularly in the presence colleagues of the same nationality. Do not be ashamed of pronouncing correctly independently of the nationality of your interlocutor.
- Enjoy the effort of using a different set of muscles in the mouth. In the beginning the "English muscles" may become stiff and even hurt, but persevere, this is only a sign of hard work.
- Not worry about having a broad or even embarrassing accent in the beginning; it doesn't matter as long as you are understood. The idea is to communicate, to say what you think or feel, and not to give a performance in speech therapy.
- Try to pronounce English words properly. As time goes by and you begin to feel relatively confident about your English, we encourage you to progressively and thoroughly study English phonetics. Bear in mind that if you keep your pronunciation as it was at the beginning you will sound like American or British people do when speaking your language with their unmistakable accent.

- Rehearse standard collocations in both conversational and radiological scenarios. Saying straightforward things such as "Do you know what I mean?" or "Would you do me a favor?" and "Who's on call today? Please would you window (and level) this image?" will provide you with extremely useful fluency tools.

Having your own *subtle* national accent in English is not a serious problem as long as the presentation conveys the correct message. However, as far as pronunciation is concerned, there are several tricky words that cannot be properly named false friends and need some extra attention.

In English there are some words that are spelled differently but sound very much the same. Consider the following, for example:

- *Ileum*: the distal portion of the small intestine, extending from the jejunum to the cecum.
- *Ilium*: the uppermost and widest of the three sections of the hip bone.

Imagine for a moment how surreal it would be for our surgeons to mix up the bowel with the hip bone. Well, I suppose you could say it could be worse – at least both anatomical structures are roughly in the same area!

Again, consider the following:

The English word *tear* means two different things according to how we pronounce it:

- If *tear* [tiar] is pronounced, we mean the watery secretion of the lacrimal glands which serves to moisten the conjunctiva.
- If *tear* [tear] is pronounced, we are referring to the action of wounding or injuring, especially by ripping apart as in "there is a longitudinal *tear* in the posterior horn of the internal meniscus".

Among the radiological words most commonly mispronounced are two which deserve a close analysis since radiologists use (or misuse) them almost every single day of their professional life. These two words are: "radiology" and "image".

Many radiologists worldwide say they are a [ra-dio-lo-gist], "I am a radiologist", instead of [rei-dio-lo-gist]. A similar difficulty occurs with intrinsically radiological words such as radiology, radiographics, radiological ... Please, from now on, avoid this unbelievably frequent mistake.

Image and *images* are two of the most commonly mispronounced radiological words. Can you imagine how many times you will say "image" or "images" in your radiological life? Please don't say [im-éich] or [im-éiches] but [ím-ich] and [ím-iches]. If you are among the vast group of radiologists who used to say [im-éich] for every single slide of every presentation, don't tell anybody and "keep on" saying [ím-ich] "as you always did". Don't worry! there are probably no records of your presentations, and if they do exist, they are not readily available.

The reason for underlining these two common mistakes is to emphasize that you have to avoid mispronunciation mistakes beginning with the most usual words in your daily practice. If you are not a chest radiologist and don't know how to pronounce, for example, "lymphangioleiomyomatosis", don't worry about this word until you have mastered the pronunciation of your day-to-day radiological terms (if you had to read out loud this weird word, you can defend yourself by saying LAM [lam] which, by the way, sounds more natural and is much more used than [lim-fan-gio-lio-maio-ma-tou-ses]).

Our piece of advice is: create a top-100 list with your day-to-day most difficult words in terms of spelling. Once you are familiar with them enlarge your list by keeping on reading out loud as many articles as you can. If you happen to be an interventional radiologist, brochures and instructions-for-use sheets can keep you posted with virtually no effort and will help you to fill in those useless time-outs between patients.

We have created a list made up of some mispronounced radiological words. Since this list is absolutely arbitrary and could vary depending on your native tongue, we encourage you to create your own list.

- Parenchyma
  Parenchyma is, in principle, an easy word to pronounce. We include it in this list because we've noticed that some lecturers, particularly Italians, tend to say [pa-ren-kái-ma].
- The letter "h"
  - "Non-pronunciation": Italian and French speakers tend to skip this letter so that when they pronounce the word "enhancement" they say [en-áns-ment] instead of [en-háns-ment]. It is true that "h" can be silent but NOT always.
  - "Over-pronunciation": Spanish doctors tend to over-pronounce the letter "h".
- Data
  Although some American radiologists say [data], the correct pronunciation of this word is [déi-ta].
- Disease/decease
  The pronunciation of *disease* can be funny since depending on how you pronounce the "s" you can be saying "decease" which is what terminal diseases end in. The correct pronunciation of *disease* is [di-ssíss] with a liquid "s"; if you say [di-sís] with a plain "s", as many Spanish and Latin American speakers do, every time you talk about, let's say, Alzheimer's disease you are talking about Alzheimer's decease or Alzheimer's death.
- Chamber
  The pronunciation of *chamber* is somewhat tricky since French speakers tend "Gallicize" it by saying [cham-bre] whereas some Spanish speakers say simply [cham-ber] instead of [cheim-ber]

- French words such as "technique"
  In English you have to say [tek-ník], "in the French way", although you say technical [ték-ni-cal].

- Hippocampus (think of *hippopotamus*)
  A lack of etymological knowledge is responsible for this tricky mistake. Many doctors worldwide say [haipo-cam-pus] as if they were talking about the hypothalamus [haipo-ta-la-mus]. Unfortunately, hippocampus has no etymological relationship to hypothalamus or hypotension. *Hippo-* means "horse" (as in *hippopotamus*) and is pronounced [hipo-cám-pus].

- Director
  Although you can say both [di-rect] and [dai-rect] only [dai-rec-tor] is correct; you cannot say [di-rec-tor].

It is beyond the scope of this manual to go over all potentially tricky words in terms of pronunciation, but we offer below a short list of more such words, and would again encourage you to create your own "personal" list.

- Medulla [me-dú-la]
- Anesthetist [a-nés-te-tist]
- Gynecology [gai-ne-có-lo-gy]
- Edema [i-di-ma]
- Case report [kéis ri-pórt, NOT kéis ré-port]
- Multidetector [multi-, NOT mul-tai]
- Oblique [o-blík, NOT o-bláik]
- Femoral [fí-mo-ral]
- Jugular [iu-gu-lar]
- Triquetrum [tri-kui-trum]

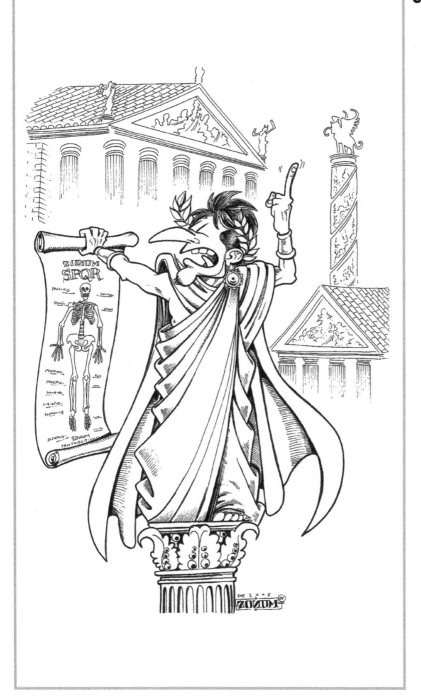

Unit IX   Latin and Greek Terminology

Introduction

Latin and Greek terminology is another obstacle to be overcome on our way to becoming fluent in medical English. Romance-language speakers (Spanish, French, Italian ...) are undoubtedly at an advantage, although this advantage can become a great drawback in terms of pronunciation and, particularly, in the use of the plural forms of Latin and Greek.

Since most Latin words used in medical English keep the Latin plural ending – e.g., metastasis, *pl.* metastases; viscus, *pl.* viscera – it is essential to understand the basis of plural rules in Latin.

All Latin nouns and adjectives have different endings for each gender (masculine, feminine, or neuter), number (singular or plural), and case – the case is a special ending that reveals the function of the word in a particular sentence. Latin adjectives must correlate with the nouns they modify in case, number, and gender. Although we can barely remember it from our days in high school, there are five different patterns of endings, each one of them is called declension.

The nominative case indicates the subject of a sentence. The genitive case denotes possession or attachment. Dropping the genitive singular ending gives the base to which the nominative plural ending is added to build the medical English plural form.

For example:

- *Corpus* (nominative singular), *corporis* (genitive singular), *corpora* (nominative plural). This is a third-declension neuter noun that means body. The corresponding forms for the accompanying adjective *callosus* are *callosum*, and *callosa*, respectively. Thus *corpus callosum* (nominative, singular, neuter), *corpora callosa* (nominative, plural, neuter).

Another example:

- *Coxa vara* (feminine singular), *coxae varae* (feminine plural), but *genu varum* (neuter, singular), *genua vara* (neuter, plural)

Table 1. The endings of Latin substantives listed by case and declension

Case	Declension							
	1st	**2nd**		**3rd**		**4th**		**5th**
	Fem.	**Masc.**	**Neut.**	**Masc./fem.**	**Neut.**	**Masc.**	**Neut.**	**Fem.**
Nominative sing.	*-a*	*-us*	*-um*	∅	∅	*-us*	*-u*	*-es*
Genitive sing.	*-ae*	*-i*	*-i*	*-is*	*-is*	*-us*	*-us*	*-ei*
Nominative pl.	*-ae*	*-i*	*-a*	*-es*	*-a*	*-us*	*-ua*	*-es*

This unit provides an extensive Latin glossary that includes the singular and plural nominative, and the genitive singular forms of each word as well as the declension and gender of each word. In some terms, additional items have been added, such as English plural endings when widely accepted (e.g., *fetus*, Latin plural *feti*, English plural *fetuses*), and Greek-origin endings kept in some Latin words (e.g., *thorax*, pl. *thoraces*, gen. *thoracos/thoracis*: chest)

The endings of Latin substantives listed by case and declension are shown in Table 1.

Examples:

- 1st declension:
  - Feminine words: *patella* (nom. sing.), *patellae* (gen.), *patellae* (nom. pl.). English *patella*.
- 2nd declension:
  - Masculine words: *humerus* (nom. sing.), *humeri* (gen.), humeri (nom. pl.). English *humerus*.
  - Neuter words: *interstitium* (nom. sing.), *interstitii* (gen.), *interstitia* (nom. pl.). English *interstice*.
- 3rd declension:
  - Masculine or feminine words: *pars* (nom. sing.), *partis* (gen.), *partes* (nom. pl.). English *part*.
  - Neuter words: *os* (nom. sing.), *oris* (gen.), *ora* (nom. pl.). English *mouth*.
- 4th declension:
  - Masculine words: *processus* (nom. sing.), *processus* (gen.), *processus* (nom. pl.). English *process*.
  - Neuter words: *cornu* (nom. sing.), *cornus* (gen.), *cornua* (nom. pl.). English *horn*.

- 5th declension:
  - Feminine words: *facies* (nom. sing.), *faciei* (gen.), *facies* (nom. pl.). English *face*.

The endings of the adjectives change according to one of these two patterns:

1. Singular: masc. *-us*, fem. *-a*, neut. *-um*. Plural: masc. *-i*, fem. *-ae*, neut. *-a*.
2. Singular: masc. *-is*, fem. *-is*, neut. *-e*. Plural: masc. *-es*, fem. *-es*, neut. *-a*.

Plural Rules

It is far from our intention to replace medical dictionaries and Latin or Greek text books. Conversely, this unit is aimed at giving some tips related to Latin and Greek terminology that can provide a consistent approach to this challenging topic.

Our first piece of advice on this subject is that whenever you write a Latin or Greek word, firstly, check its spelling and, secondly, if the word you want to write is a plural one, never make it up. Although guessing the plural form could be acceptable as an exercise in itself, double-check the word by looking it up in a medical dictionary.

The following plural rules are useful to at least give us self-confidence in the use of usual Latin or Greek terms such as *metastasis – metastases, pelvis – pelves, bronchus – bronchi*, etc. ...

Some overseas doctors do think that *metastasis* and *metastases* are equivalent terms, and they are absolutely wrong; the difference between a unique liver metastasis and multiple liver metastases is so obvious that no additional comment is needed.

There are many Latin and Greek words whose singular forms are almost never used as well as Latin and Greek terms whose plural forms are seldom said or written. Let us think, for example, about the singular form of *viscera* (*viscus*). Very few physicians are aware that the liver is a *viscus* whereas the liver and spleen are *viscera*. From a colloquial standpoint this discussion might be considered futile, but those who write papers do know that Latin/Greek terminology is always a nightmare and needs thorough revision, and that terms seldom used on a day-to-day basis have to be properly written in a scientific article. Again, let us consider the plural form of *pelvis* (*pelves*). To talk about several pelves is so rare that many doctors have never wondered what the plural form of pelvis is.

Although there are some exceptions, the following general rules can be helpful with plural terms:

- Words ending in *-us* change to *-i* (2nd declension masculine words):
  - *bronchus – bronchi*

- Words ending in -*um* change to -*a* (2nd declension neuter words):
  - *acetabulum* – *acetabula*

- Words ending in -*a* change to -*ae* (1st declension feminine words):
  - *vena* – *venae*

- Words ending in -*ma* change to -*mata* or -*mas* (3rd declension neuter words of Greek origin):
  - *sarcoma* – *sarcomata/sarcomas*

- Words ending in -*is* change to -*es* (3rd declension masculine or feminine words):
  - *metastasis* – *metastases*

- Words ending in -*itis* change to -*itides* (3rd declension masculine or feminine words):
  - *arthritis* – *arthritides*

- Words ending in -*x* change to -*ces* (3rd declension masculine or feminine words):
  - *pneumothorax* – *pneumothoraces*

- Words ending in -*cyx* change to -*cyges* (3rd declension masculine or feminine words):
  - *coccyx* – *coccyges*

- Words ending in -*ion* change to -*ia* (2nd declension neuter words, most of Greek origin):
  - *criterion* – *criteria*

List of Latin and Greek Terms and Their Plurals

Abbreviations:

adj.   adjective
Engl. English
fem.   feminine
gen.   genitive
Gr.   Greek
Lat.   Latin
lit.   literally
m.   muscle
masc. masculine
neut. neuter
pl.   plural
sing. singular

A

- **Abdomen**, pl. **abdomina**, gen. **abdominis**. Abdomen. 3rd declension neut.
- **Abducens**, pl. **abducentes**, gen. **abducentis** (from the verb *abduco*, to detach, to lead away). 3rd declension.
- **Abductor**, pl. **abductores**, gen. **abductoris** (from the verb *abduco*, to detach, to lead away). 3rd declension masc.
- **Acetabulum**, pl. **acetabula**, gen. **acetabuli**. Cotyle. 2nd declension neut.
- **Acinus**, pl. **acini**, gen. **acini**. Acinus. 2nd declension masc.
- **Adductor**, pl. **adductores**, gen. **adductoris**. Adductor. 3rd declension masc.
- **Aditus**, pl. **aditus**, gen. **aditus**. Entrance to a cavity. 4th declension masc.
  – *Aditus ad antrum, aditus glottidis inferior*, etc.
- **Agger**, pl. **aggeres**, gen. **aggeris**. Prominence. 3rd declension masc.
  – *Agger valvae venae, agger nasi, agger perpendicularis*, etc.
- **Ala**, pl. **alae**, gen. **alae**. Wing. 1st declension fem.
- **Alveolus**, pl. **alveoli**, gen. **alveoli**. Alveolus (lit. *basin*). 2nd declension masc.
- **Alveus**, pl. **alvei**, gen. **alvei**. Cavity, hollow. 2nd declension masc.
- **Amoeba**, pl. **amoebae**, gen. **amoebae**. Ameba. 1st declension fem.
- **Ampulla**, pl. **ampullae**, gen. **ampullae**. Ampoule, blister. 1st declension fem.
- **Anastomosis**, pl. **anastomoses**, gen. **anastomosis**. Anastomosis. 3rd declension.
- **Angulus**, pl. **anguli**, gen. **anguli**. Angle, apex, corner. 2nd declension neut.
- **Annulus**, pl. **annuli**, gen. **annuli**. Ring. 2nd declension masc.
- **Ansa**, pl. **ansae**, gen. **ansae**. Loop, hook, handle. 1st declension fem.
- **Anterior**, pl. **anteriores**, gen. **anterioris**. Foremost, that is before, former. 3rd declension masc.
- **Antrum**, pl. **antra**, gen. **antri**. Antrum, hollow, cave. 2nd declension neut.
- **Anus**, pl. **ani**, gen. **ani**. Anus (lit. *ring*). 2nd declension masc.
- **Aorta**, pl. **Aortae**, gen. **aortae**. Aorta. 1st declension fem.
- **Apex**, pl. **apices**, gen. **apices**. Apex (top, summit, cap). 3rd declension masc.
- **Aphtha**, pl. **aphthae**, gen. **aphthae**. Aphtha (small ulcer). 1st declension fem.
- **Aponeurosis**, pl. **aponeuroses**, gen. **aponeurosis**. Aponeurosis. 3rd declension.
- **Apophysis**, pl. **apophyses**, gen. **apophysos/apophysis**. Apophysis. 3rd declension fem.
- **Apparatus**, pl. **apparatus**, gen. **apparatus**. Apparatus, system. 4th declension masc.
- **Appendix**, pl. **appendices**, gen. **appendicis**. Appendage. 3rd declension fem.
- **Area**, pl. **areae**, gen. **areae**. Area. 1st declension fem.

- **Areola**, pl. **areolae**, gen. **areolae**. Areola (lit. *little area*). 1st declension fem.
- **Arrector**, pl. **arrectores**, gen. **arrectoris**. Erector, tilt upwards. 3rd declension masc.
- **Arteria**, pl. **arteriae**, gen. **arteriae**. Artery. 1st declension fem.
- **Arteriola**, pl. **arteriolae**, gen. **arteriolae**. Arteriola (small artery). 1st declension fem.
- **Arthritis**, pl. **arthritides**, gen. **arthritidis**. Arthritis. 3rd declension fem.
- **Articularis**, pl. **articulares**, gen. **articularis**. Articular, affecting the joints. 3rd declension masc. (adj.: masc. *articularis*, fem. *articularis*, neut. *articulare*).
- **Articulatio**, pl. **articulationes**, gen. **articulationis**. Joint. 3rd declension fem.
- **Atlas**, pl. **atlantes**, gen. **atlantis**. First cervical vertebra. 3rd declension masc.
- **Atrium**, pl. **atria**, gen. **atrii**. Atrium. 2nd declension neut.
- **Auricula**, pl. **auriculae**, gen. **auriculae**. Auricula (ear flap). Auricular (auricular appendix of the cardiac atrium). 1st declension fem.
- **Auricularis m.**, pl. **auriculares**, gen. **auricularis**. Pertaining to the ear. 3rd declension masc.
- **Auris**, pl. **aures**, gen. **auris**. Ear. 3rd declension fem.
- **Axilla**, pl. **axillae**, gen. **axillae**. Armpit. 1st declension fem.
- **Axis**, pl. **axes**, gen. **axis**. Second cervical vertebra, axis. 3rd declension masc.

B
- **Bacillus**, pl. **bacilli**, gen. **bacilli**. Stick-shape bacterium (lit. *small stick*). 2nd declension masc.
- **Bacterium**, pl. **bacteria**, gen. **bacterii**. Bacterium. 2nd declension neut.
- **Basis**, pl. **bases**, gen. **basis**. Basis, base. 3rd declension fem.
- **Biceps m.**, pl. **bicipites**, gen. **bicipitis**. A muscle with two heads. 3rd declension masc.
  - Biceps + genitive. Biceps *brachii* (*brachium*, arm)
- **Borborygmus**, pl. **borborygmi**, gen. **borborygmi**. Borborygmus (gastrointestinal sound). 2nd declension masc.
- **Brachium**, pl. **brachia**, gen. **brachii**. Arm. 2nd declension neut.
- **Brevis**, pl. **breves**, gen. **brevis**. Short, little, small. 3rd declension masc. (adj.: masc. *brevis*, fem. *brevis*, neut. *breve*).
- **Bronchium**, pl. **bronchia**, gen. **bronchii**. Bronchus. 2nd declension neut.
- **Buccinator m.**, pl. **buccinatores**, gen. **buccinatoris**. Buccinator m. (trumpeter's muscle). 3rd declension masc.
- **Bulla**, pl. **bullae**, gen. **bullae**. Bulla. 1st declension fem.
- **Bursa**, pl. **bursae**, gen. **bursae**. Bursa (bag, pouch). 1st declension fem.

C

- **Caecum**, pl. **caeca**, gen. **caeci**. Blind. 2nd declension neut. (adj.: masc. *caecus*, fem. *caeca*, neut. *caecum*).
- **Calcaneus**, pl. **calcanei**, gen. **calcanei**. Calcaneus (from *calx*, heel). 2nd declension masc.
- **Calculus**, pl. **calculi**, gen. **calculi**. Stone (lit. *pebble*). 2nd declension masc.
- **Calix**, pl. **calices**, gen. **calicis**. Calix (lit. *cup, goblet*). 3rd declension masc.
- **Calx**, pl. **calces**, gen. **calcis**. Heel. 3rd declension masc.
- **Canalis**, pl. **canales**, gen. **canalis**. Channel, conduit. 3rd declension masc.
- **Cancellus**, pl. **cancelli**, gen. **cancelli**. Reticulum, lattice, grid. 2nd declension masc.
- **Cancer**, pl. **cancera**, gen. **canceri**. Cancer. 3rd declension neut.
- **Capillus**, pl. **capilli**, gen. **capilli**. Hair. 2nd declension masc.
- **Capitatus**, pl. **capitati**, gen. **capitati**. Capitate, having or forming a head. 2nd declension masc. (adj.: masc. *capitatus*, fem. *capitata*, neut. *capitatum*).
- **Capitulum**, pl. **capitula**, gen. **capituli**. Head of a structure, condyle. 2nd declension neut.
- **Caput**, pl. **capita**, gen. **capitis**. Head. 3rd declension neut.
- **Carcinoma**, pl. Lat. **carcinomata**, pl. Engl. **carcinomas**, gen. **carcinomatis**. Carcinoma (epithelial cancer). 3rd declension neut.
- **Carina**, pl. **carinae**, gen. **carinae**. Carina (lit. *keel, bottom of ship*). 1st declension fem.
- **Cartilago**, pl. **cartilagines**, gen. **cartilaginis**. Cartilage. 3rd declension neut.
- **Cauda**, pl. **caudae**, gen. **caudae**. Tail. 1st declension fem.
  - *Cauda equina* (adj.: masc. *equinus*, fem. *equina*, neut. *equinum*. Concerning horses).
- **Caverna**, pl. **cavernae**, gen. **cavernae**. Cavern. 1st declension fem.
- **Cavitas**, pl. **cavitates**, gen. **cavitatis**. Cavity. 3rd declension fem.
- **Cavum**, pl. **cava**, gen. **cavi**. Cavum (hole, pit, depression). 2nd declension neut.
- **Cella**, pl. **cellae**, gen. **cellae**. Cell (lit. *cellar, wine storeroom*). 1st declension fem.
- **Centrum**, pl. **centra**, gen. **centri**. Center. 2nd declension neut.
- **Cerebellum**, pl. **cerebella**, gen. **cerebelli**. Cerebellum. 2nd declension neut.
- **Cerebrum**, pl. **cerebra**, gen. **cerebri**. Brain. 2nd declension neut.
- **Cervix**, pl. **cervices**, gen. **cervicis**. Neck. 3rd declension fem.
- **Chiasma**, pl. **chiasmata**, gen. **chiasmatis/chiasmatos**. Chiasm. 3rd declension neut.
- **Choana**, pl. **choanae**, gen. **choanae**. Choana. 1st declension fem.
  - *Choanae narium* (*naris*, gen. sing. *naris*, gen. pl. *narium*, nose). Posterior opening of the nasal fossae.

- **Chorda**, pl. **chordae**, gen. **chordae**. String. 1st declension fem.
  - *Chorda tympani*. A nerve given off from the facial nerve in the facial canal that crosses over the tympanic membrane (*tympanum*, gen. *tympani*. Eardrum).
- **Chorion**, pl. **choria**, gen. **chorii**. Chorion (membrane enclosing the fetus). 2nd declension neut.
- **Cicatrix**, pl. **cicatrices**, gen. **cicatricis**. Scar. 3rd declension fem.
- **Cilium**, pl. **cilia**, gen. **cilii**. Cilium (lit. *upper eyelid*). 2nd declension neut.
- **Cingulum**, pl. **cingula**, gen. **cinguli**. Cingulum (belt-shaped structure, lit. *belt*). 2nd declension neut.
- **Cisterna**, pl. **cisternae**, gen. **cisternae**. Cistern. 1st declension fem.
- **Claustrum**, pl. **claustra**, gen. **claustri**. Claustrum. 2nd declension neut.
- **Clitoris**, pl. **clitorides**, gen. **clitoridis**. Clitoris. 3rd declension.
- **Clivus**, pl. **clivi**, gen. **clivi**. Clivus (part of the skull, lit. *slope*). 2nd declension masc.
- **Clostridium**, pl. **clostridia**, gen. **clostridii**. Clostridium (genus of bacteria). 2nd declension neut.
- **Coccus**, pl. **cocci**, gen. **cocci**. Coccus (rounded bacterium, lit. *a scarlet dye*). 2nd declension masc.
- **Coccyx**, pl. **coccyges**, gen. **coccygis**. Coccyx. 3rd declension masc.
- **Cochlea**, pl. **cochleae**, gen. **cochleae**. Cochlea (lit. *snail shell*). 1st declension fem.
- **Collum**, pl. **colla**, gen. **colli**. Neck. 2nd declension neut.
- **Comedo**, pl. **comedones**, gen. **comedonis**. Comedo (a dilated hair follicle filled with keratin). 3rd declension masc.
- **Comunis**, pl. **comunes**, gen. **comunis**. Common. 3rd declension masc. (adj.: masc./fem. *comunis*, neut. *comune*).
- **Concha**, pl. **conchae**, gen. **conchae**. Concha (shell-shaped structure). 1st declension fem.
- **Condyloma**, pl. **condylomata**, gen. **condylomatis**. Condyloma. 3rd declension neut.
  - *Condyloma acuminatum*.
- **Conjunctiva**, pl. **conjunctivae**, gen. **conjunctivae**. Conjunctiva. 1st declension fem.
- **Constrictor**, pl. **constrictores**, gen. **constrictoris**. Sphincter. 3rd declension masc.
- **Conus**, pl. **coni**, gen. **coni**. Cone. 2nd declension masc.
  - *Conus medullaris* (from *medulla*, pl. *medullae*. The tapering end of the spinal cord).
- **Cor**, pl. **corda**, gen. **cordis**. Heart. 3rd declension neut.
- **Corium**, pl. **coria**, gen. **corii**. Dermis (lit. *skin*). 2nd declension neut.
- **Cornu**, pl. **cornua**, gen. **cornus**. Horn. 4th declension neut.
- **Corona**, pl. **coronae**, gen. **coronae**. Corona (lit. *crown*). 1st declension fem.
  - *Corona radiata*, pl. *coronae radiatae*, gen. *coronae radiatae*.

- **Corpus**, pl. **corpora**, gen. **corporis**. Body. 3rd declension neut.
  - *Corpus callosum, corpus cavernosum.*
- **Corpusculum**, pl. **corpuscula**, gen. **corpusculi**. Corpuscle. 2nd declension neut.
- **Cortex**, pl. **cortices**, gen. **corticis**. Cortex, outer covering. 3rd declension masc.
- **Coxa**, pl. **coxae**, gen. **coxae**. Hip. 1st declension fem.
- **Cranium**, pl. **crania**, gen. **cranii**. Skull. 2nd declension neut.
- **Crisis**, pl. **crises**, gen. **crisos/crisis**. Crisis. 3rd declension fem.
- **Crista**, pl. **cristae**, gen. **cristae**. Crest. 1st declension fem.
  - *Crista galli* (from *gallus*, pl. *galli*, rooster). The midline process of the ethmoid bone arising from the cribriform plate.
- **Crus**, pl. **crura**, gen. **cruris**. Leg, leg-like structure. 3rd declension neut.
  - *Crura diaphragmatis.*
- **Crusta**, pl. **crustae**, gen. **crustae**. Crust, hard surface. 1st declension fem.
- **Crypta**, pl. **cryptae**, gen. **cryptae**. Crypt. 1st declension fem.
- **Cubitus**, pl. **cubiti**, gen. **cubiti**. Ulna (lit. *forearm*). 2nd declension masc.
- **Cubitus**, pl. **cubitus**, gen. **cubitus**. State of lying down. 4th declension masc.
  - *De cubito supino/prono.*
- **Culmen**, pl. **culmina**, gen. **culminis**. Peak, top. Top of cerebellar lobe. 3rd declension neut.
- **Cuneiforme**, pl. **cuneiformia**, gen. **cuneiformis**. Wedge-shaped structure. 3rd declension neut. (adj.: masc. *cuneiformis*, fem. *cuneiformis*, neut. *cuneiforme*).

D

- **Decussatio**, pl. **decussationes**, gen. **decussationis**. Decussation. 3rd declension fem.
- **Deferens**, pl. **deferentes**, gen. **deferentis**. Spermatic duct (from the verb *defero*, to carry). 3rd declension masc.
- **Dens**, pl. **dentes**, gen. **dentis**. Tooth. 3rd declension masc.
- **Dermatitis**, pl. **dermatitides**, gen. **dermatitis**. Dermatitis. 3rd declension.
- **Dermatosis**, pl. **dermatoses**, gen. **dermatosis**. Dermatosis. 3rd declension.
- **Diaphragma**, pl. **diaphragmata**, gen. **diaphragmatis**. Diaphragm. 3rd declension neut.
- **Diaphysis**, pl. **diaphyses**, gen. **diaphysis**. Shaft. 3rd declension.
- **Diarthrosis**, pl. **diarthroses**, gen. **diarthrosis**. Diarthrosis. 3rd declension.
- **Diastema**, pl. **diastemata**, gen. **diastematis**. Diastema (congenital fissure). 3rd declension.
- **Digastricus m.**, pl. **digastrici**, gen. **digastrici**. Digastric (having two bellies). 2nd declension masc.

- **Digitus**, pl. **digiti**, gen. sing. **digiti**, gen. pl. **digitorum**. Finger. 2nd declension masc.
  - *Extensor digiti minimi, flexor superficialis digitorum.*
- **Diverticulum**, pl. **diverticula**, gen. **diverticuli**. Diverticulum. 2nd declension neut.
- **Dorsum**, pl. **dorsa**, gen. **dorsi**. Back. 2nd declension neut.
- **Ductus**, pl. **ductus**, gen. **ductus**. Duct. 4th declension masc.
  - *Ductus arteriosus, ductus deferens.*
- **Duodenum**, pl. **duodena**, gen. **duodeni**. Duodenum (lit. *twelve*. The duodenum measures 12 times a finger). 2nd declension neut.

E
- **Ecchymosis**, pl. **ecchymoses**, gen. **ecchymosis**. Ecchymosis. 3rd declension.
- **Effluvium**, pl. **effluvia**, gen. **effluvii**. Effluvium (fall). 2nd declension neut.
- **Encephalitis**, pl. **encephalitides**, gen. **encephalitidis**. Encephalitis. 3rd declension fem.
- **Endocardium**, pl. **endocardia**, gen. **endocardii**. Endocardium. 2nd declension neut.
- **Endometrium**, pl. **endometria**, gen. **endometrii**. Endometrium. 2nd declension neut.
- **Endothelium**, pl. **endothelia**, gen. **endothelii**. Endothelium. 2nd declension neut.
- **Epicondylus**, pl. **epicondyli**, gen. **epicondyli**. Epicondylus. 2nd declension masc.
- **Epidermis**, pl. **epidermides**, gen. **epidermidis**. Epidermis. 3rd declension.
- **Epididymis**, pl. **epididymes**, gen. **epididymis**. Epididymis. 3rd declension.
- **Epiphysis**, pl. **epiphyses**, gen. **epiphysis**. Epiphysis. 3rd declension.
- **Epithelium**, pl. **epithelia**, gen. **epithelii**. Epithelium. 2nd declension neut.
- **Esophagus**, pl. **esophagi**, gen. **esophagi**. Esophagus. 2nd declension masc.
- **Exostosis**, pl. **exostoses**, gen. **exostosis**. Exostosis. 3rd declension.
- **Extensor**, pl. **extensores**, gen. **extensoris**. A muscle the contraction of which stretches out a structure. 3rd declension masc.
  - *Extensor carpi ulnaris m., extensor digitorum communis m., extensor hallucis longus/brevis m.*, etc.
- **Externus**, pl. **externi**, gen. **externi**. External, outward. 2nd declension masc (adj.: masc. *externus*, fem. *externa*, gen. *externum*).

F

- **Facies**, pl. **facies**, gen. **faciei**. Face. 5th declension fem.
- **Falx**, pl. **falces**, gen. **falcis**. Sickle-shaped structure. 3rd declension fem.
  - *Falx cerebrii.*
- **Fascia**, pl. **fasciae**, gen. **fasciae**. Fascia. 1st declension fem.
- **Fasciculus**, pl. **fasciculi**, gen. **fasciculi**. Fasciculus. 2nd declension masc.
- **Femur**, pl. **femora**, gen. **femoris**. Femur. 3rd declension neut.
- **Fenestra**, pl. **fenestrae**, gen. **fenestrae**. Window, hole. 1st declension fem.
- **Fetus**, Lat. pl. **feti/fetus**, Eng. pl. **fetuses**, gen. **feti/fetus**. Fetus. 2nd declension masc/4th declension masc.
- **Fibra**, pl. **fibrae**, gen. **fibrae**. Fiber. 1st declension fem.
- **Fibula**, pl. **fibulae**, gen. **fibulae**. Fibula. 1st declension fem.
- **Filamentum**, pl. **filamenta**, gen. **filamentii**. Filament. 2nd declension neut.
- **Filaria**, pl. **filariae**, gen. **filariae**. Filaria. 1st declension fem.
- **Filum**, pl. **fila**, gen. **fili**. Filamentous structure. 2nd declension neut.
  - *Filum terminale*
- **Fimbria**, pl. **fimbriae**, gen. **fimbriae**. Fimbria (lit. *fringe*). 1st declension fem.
- **Fistula**, pl. **fistulae**, gen. **fistulae**. Fistula (lit. *pipe, tube*). 1st declension fem.
- **Flagellum**, pl. **flagella**, gen. **flagelli**. Flagellum (whip-like locomotory organelle). 2nd declension neut.
- **Flexor**, pl. **flexores**, gen. **flexoris**. A muscle whose action flexes a joint. 3rd declension masc.
  - *Flexor carpi radialis/ulnaris mm., flexor pollicis longus/brevis mm.,* etc.
- **Flexura**, pl. **flexurae**, gen. **flexurae**. Flexure, curve, bow. 1st declension fem.
- **Folium**, pl. **folia**, gen. **folii**. Leaf-shaped structure (lit. *leaf*). 2nd declension neut.
- **Folliculus**, pl. **folliculi**, gen. **folliculi**. Follicle. 2nd declension masc.
- **Foramen**, pl. **foramina**, gen. **foraminis**. Foramen, hole. 3rd declension neut.
  - *Foramen rotundum, foramen ovale.*
  - *Foramina cribrosa*, pl. (multiple pores in lamina cribrosa).
- **Formula**, pl. **formulae**, gen. **formulae**. Formula. 1st declension fem.
- **Fornix**, pl. **fornices**, gen. **fornicis**. Fornix (arch-shaped structure). 3rd declension masc.
- **Fossa**, pl. **fossae**, gen. **fossae**. Fossa, depression. 1st declension fem.
- **Fovea**, pl. **foveae**, gen. **foveae**. Fovea, depression, pit. 1st declension fem.
- **Frenulum**, pl. **frenula**, gen. **frenuli**. Bridle-like structure. 2nd declension neut.
- **Fungus**, pl. **fungi**, gen. **fungi**. Fungus (lit. *mushroom*). 2nd declension masc.
- **Funiculus**, pl. **funiculi**, gen. **funiculi**. Cord, string. 2nd declension masc.

- **Furfur,** pl. **furfures,** gen. **furfuris.** Dandruff. 3rd declension masc.
- **Furunculus,** pl. **furunculi,** gen. **furunculi.** Furuncle. 2nd declension masc.

G

- **Galea,** pl. **galeae,** gen. **galeae.** Cover, a structure shaped like a helmet (lit. *helmet*). 1st declension fem.
  - *Galea aponeurotica,* pl. *galeae aponeuroticae* (epicranial aponeurosis).
- **Ganglion,** pl. **ganglia,** gen. **ganglii.** Node. 2nd declension masc.
- **Geniculum,** pl. **genicula,** gen. **geniculi.** Geniculum (knee-shaped structure). 2nd declension neut.
- **Geniohyoideus m.,** pl. **geniohyoidei,** gen. **geniohyoidei.** Glenohyoid muscle. 2nd declension masc.
- **Genu,** pl. **genua,** gen. **genus.** Knee. 4th declension neut.
- **Genus,** pl. **genera,** gen. **generis.** Gender. 3rd declension neut.
- **Gestosis,** pl. **gestoses,** gen. **gestosis.** Gestosis (pregnancy impairment). 3rd declension.
- **Gingiva,** pl. **gingivae,** gen. **gingivae.** Gum. 1st declension fem.
- **Glabella,** pl. **glabellae,** gen. **glabellae.** Small lump/mass. 1st declension fem.
- **Glandula,** pl. **glandulae,** gen. **glandulae.** Gland. 1st declension fem.
- **Glans,** pl. **glandes,** gen. **glandis.** Glans (lit. *acorn*). 3rd declension fem.
  - *Glans penis.*
- **Globus,** pl. **globi,** gen. **globi.** Globus, round body. 2nd declension masc.
- **Glomerulus,** pl. **glomeruli,** gen. **glomeruli.** Glomerule. 2nd declension masc.
- **Glomus,** pl. **glomera,** gen. **glomeris.** Glomus (ball-shaped body). 3rd declension.
- **Glottis,** pl. **glottides,** gen. **glottidis.** Glottis. 3rd declension.
- **Gluteus m.,** pl. **glutei,** gen. **glutei.** Buttock. 2nd declension masc.
- **Gracilis m.,** pl. **graciles,** gen. **gracilis.** Graceful. 3rd declension masc (adj.: masc. *gracilis,* fem. *gracilis,* neut. *gracile*).
- **Granulatio,** pl. **granulationes,** gen. **granulationis.** Granulation. 3rd declension.
- **Gumma,** pl. **gummata,** gen. **gummatis.** Syphiloma. 3rd declension neut.
- **Gutta,** pl. **guttae,** gen. **guttae.** Gout. 1st declension fem.
- **Gyrus,** pl. **gyri,** gen. **gyri.** Convolution. 2nd declension masc.
- **Gastrocnemius m.,** pl. **gastrocnemii,** gen. **gastrocnemii.** Calf muscle. 2nd declension masc.

H

- **Hallux,** pl. **halluces,** gen. **hallucis.** First toe. 3rd declension masc.
- **Hamatus,** pl. **hamati,** gen. **hamati.** Hamate bone. 2nd declension masc. (adj.: masc. *hamatus,* fem. *hamata,* neut. *hamatum.* Hooked).
- **Hamulus,** pl. **hamuli,** gen. **hamuli.** Hamulus (lit. *small hook*). 2nd declension masc.

- **Haustrum**, pl. **haustra**, gen. **haustri**. Pouch from the lumen of the colon. 2nd declension neut.
- **Hiatus**, pl. **hiatus**, gen. **hiatus**. Gap, cleft. 4th declension masc.
- **Hilum**, pl. **hila**, gen. **hili**. Hilum (the part of an organ where the neurovascular bundle enters). 2nd declension neut.
- **Hircus**, pl. **hirci**, gen. **hirci**. Hircus (armpit hair, lit. *goat*). 2nd declension masc.
- **Humerus**, pl. **humeri**, gen. **humeri**. Humerus. 2nd declension masc.
- **Humor**, pl. **humores**, gen. **humoris**. Humor, fluid. 3rd declension masc.
- **Hypha**, pl. **hyphae**, gen. **hyphae**. Hypha, tubular cell (lit. Gr. *web*). 1st declension fem.
- **Hypophysis**, pl. **hypophyses**, gen. **hypophysis**. Pituitary gland (lit. *undergrowth*). 3rd declension.
- **Hypothenar**, pl. **hypothenares**, gen. **hypothenaris**. Hypothenar (from Gr. *thenar*, the palm of the hand). 3rd declension.

I

- **Ilium**, pl. **ilia**, gen. **ilii**. Iliac bone. 2nd declension neut.
- **In situ**. In position (from *situs*, pl. *situs*, gen. *situs*, site). 4th declension masc.
- **Incisura**, pl. **incisurae**, gen. **incisurae**. Incisure (from the verb *incido*, cut into). 1st declension fem.
- **Incus**, pl. **incudes**, gen. **incudis**. Incus (lit. *anvil*). 3rd declension fem.
- **Index**, pl. **indices**, gen. **indicis**. Index (second digit, forefinger), guide. 3rd declension masc.
- **Indusium**, pl. **indusia**, gen. **indusii**. Indusium (membrane, amnion). 2nd declension neut.
- **Inferior**, pl. **inferiores**, gen. **inferioris**. Inferior. 3rd declension masc.
- **Infundibulum**, pl. **infundibula**, gen. **infundibuli**. Infundibulum. 2nd declension neut.
- **Insula**, pl. **insulae**, gen. **insulae**. Insula. 1st declension fem.
- **Intermedius**, pl. **intermedii**, gen. **intermedii**. In the middlle of. 2nd declension masc. (adj.: masc. *intermedius*, fem. *intermedia*, neut. *intermedium*)
- **Internus**, pl. **interni**, gen. **interni**. Internal. 2nd declension masc. (adj.: masc. *internus*, fem. *interna*, neut. *internum*).
- **Interosseus**, gen. **interossei**, pl. **interossei**. Interosseous. 2nd declension masc. (adj.: masc. *interosseus*, fem. *interossea*, neut. *interosseum*).
- **Intersectio**, pl. **intersectiones**, gen. **intersectionis**. Intersection. 3rd declension fem.
- **Interstitium**, pl. **interstitia**, gen. **interstitii**. Interstice. 2nd declension neut.
- **Intestinum**, pl. **intestina**, gen. **intestini**. Bowel. 2nd declension neut.
- **Iris**, pl. **irides**, gen. **iridis**. Iris. 3rd declension masc.
- **Ischium**, pl. **ischia**, gen. **ischii**. Ischium. 2nd declension neut.

- **Isthmus**, pl. Lat. **isthmi**, pl. Engl. **isthmuses**, gen. **isthmi**. Constriction, narrrow passage. 2nd declension masc.

J

- **Jejunum**, pl. **jejuna**, gen. **jejuni**. Jejunum (from Lat. adj. *jejunus*, fasting, empty). 2nd declension neut.
- **Jugular**, pl. **jugulares**, gen. **jugularis**. Jugular vein (lit. relating to the throat, from Lat. *jugulus*, throat). 3rd declension.
- **Junctura**, pl. **juncturae**, gen. **juncturae**. Joint, junction. 1st declension fem.

L

- **Labium**, pl. **labia**, gen. **labii**. Lip. 2nd declension neut.
- **Labrum**, pl. **labra**, gen. **labri**. Rim, edge, lip. 2nd declension neut.
- **Lacuna**, pl. **lacunae**, gen. **lacunae**. Pond, pit, hollow. 1st declension fem.
- **Lamellipodium**, pl. **lamellipodia**, gen. **lamellipodii**. Lamellipodium. 2nd declension neut.
- **Lamina**, pl. **laminae**, gen. **laminae**. Layer. 1st declension fem.
  - *Lamina papyracea, lamina perpendicularis.*
- **Larva**, pl. **larvae**, gen. **larvae**. Larva. 1st declension fem.
- **Larynx**, pl. Lat. **larynges**, pl. Engl. **larynxes**, gen. **laryngis**. Larynx. 3rd declension.
- **Lateralis**, pl. **laterales**, gen. **lateralis**. Lateral. 3rd declension masc. (adj.: masc. *lateralis*, fem. *lateralis*, neut. *laterale*).
- **Latissimus**, pl. **latissimi**, gen. **latissimi**. Very wide, the widest. 2nd declension masc. (adj.: masc. *latissimus*, fem. *latissima*, neut. *latissimum*).
- **Latus**, pl. **latera**, gen. **lateris**. Flank. 3rd declension neut.
- **Latus**, pl. **lati**, gen. **lati**. Wide, broad. 2nd declension masc. (adj.: masc. *latus*, fem. *lata*, neut. *latum*).
- **Lemniscus**, pl. **lemnisci**, gen. **lemnisci**. Lemniscus (lit. *ribbon*). 2nd declension masc.
- **Lentigo**, pl. **lentigines**, gen. **lentiginis**. Lentigo (lit. *lentil-shaped spot*). 3rd declension.
- **Levator**, pl. **levatores**, gen. **levatoris**. Lifter (from Lat. verb *levo*, to lift). 3rd declension masc.
- **Lien**, pl. **lienes**, gen. **lienis**. Spleen. 3rd declension masc.
- **Lienculus**, pl. **lienculi**, gen. **lienculi**. Accessory spleen. 2nd declension masc.
- **Ligamentum**, pl. **ligamenta**, gen. **ligamenti**. Ligament. 2nd declension neut.
- **Limbus**, pl. **limbi**, gen. **limbi**. Border, edge. 2nd declension masc.
- **Limen**, pl. **limina**, gen. **liminis**. Threshold. 3rd declension neut.
- **Linea**, pl. **lineae**, gen. **lineae**. Line. 1st declension fem.
- **Lingua**, pl. **linguae**, gen. **linguae**. Tongue. 1st declension fem.
- **Lingualis**, pl. **linguales**, gen. **lingualis**. Relative to the tongue. 3rd declension masc. (adj.: masc. *lingualis*, fem. *lingualis*, neut. *linguale*).

- **Lingula**, pl. **lingulae**, gen. **lingulae**. Lingula (tongue-shaped). 1st declension fem.
- **Liquor**, pl. **liquores**, gen. **liquoris**. Fluid. 3rd declension masc.
- **Lobulus**, pl. **lobuli**, gen. **lobuli**. Lobule. 2nd declension masc.
- **Lobus**, pl. **lobi**, gen. **lobi**. Lobe. 2nd declension masc.
- **Loculus**, pl. **loculi**, gen. **loculi**. Loculus (small chamber). 2nd declension masc.
- **Locus**, pl. **loci**, gen. **loci**. Locus (place, position, point). 2nd declension masc.
- **Longissimus**, pl. **longissimi**, gen. **longissimi**. Very long, the longest. 2nd declension masc. (Adj masc. longissimus, fem. longissima, neut. longissimum).
  - *Longissimus dorsi/capitis mm.* (long muscle of the back/head)
- **Longus**, pl. **longi**, gen. **longi**. Long. 2nd declension masc. (adj.: masc. *longus*, fem. *longa*, neut. *longum*).
  - *Longus colli m.* (long muscle of the neck).
- **Lumbar**, pl. **lumbares**, gen. **lumbaris**. Lumbar. 3rd declension.
- **Lumbus**, pl. **lumbi**, gen. **lumbi**. Loin. 2nd declension masc.
- **Lumen**, pl. **lumina**, gen. **luminis**. Lumen. 3rd declension neut.
- **Lunatum**, pl. **lunata**, gen. **lunati**. Lunate bone, crescent-shaped structure. 2nd declension neut. (adj.: masc. *lunatus*, fem. *lunata*, neut. *lunatum*).
- **Lunula**, pl. **lunulae**, gen. **lunulae**. Lunula. 1st declension fem.
- **Lymphonodus**, pl. **lymphonodi**, gen. **lymphonodi**. Lymph node. 2nd declension masc.

M

- **Macula**, pl. **maculae**, gen. **maculae**. Macula, spot. 1st declension fem.
- **Magnus**, pl. **magni**, gen. **magni**. Large, great. 2nd declension masc. (adj.: masc. *magnus*, fem. *magna*, neut. *magnum*).
- **Major**, pl. **majores**, gen. **majoris**. Greater. 3rd declension masc./fem.
- **Malleollus**, pl. **malleoli**, gen. **malleoli**. Malleollus (lit. *small hammer*). 2nd declension masc.
- **Malleus**, pl. **mallei**, gen. **mallei**. Malleus (lit. *hammer*). 2nd declension masc.
- **Mamilla**, pl. **mamillae**, gen. **mamillae**. Mamilla. 1st declension fem.
- **Mamma**, pl. **mammae**, gen. **mammae**. Breast. 1st declension fem.
- **Mandibula**, pl. **mandibulae**, gen. **mandibulae**. Jaw. 1st declension fem.
- **Mandibular**, pl. **mandibulares**, gen. **mandibularis**. Relative to the jaw. 3rd declension.
- **Manubrium**, pl. **manubria**, gen. **manubrii**. Manubrium (lit. *handle*). 2nd declension neut.
  - *Manubrium sterni*, pl. *manubria sterna* (superior part of the sternum).
- **Manus**, pl. **manus**, gen. **manus**. Hand. 4th declension fem.
- **Margo**, pl. **margines**, gen. **marginis**. Margin. 3rd declension fem.
- **Matrix**, pl. **matrices**, gen. **matricis**. Matrix (formative portion of a structure, surrounding substance). 3rd declension fem.

- **Maxilla**, pl. **maxillae**, gen. **maxillae**. Maxilla. 1st declension fem.
- **Maximus**, pl. **maximi**, gen. **maximi**. The greatest, the biggest, the largest. 2nd declension masc. (adj.: masc. *maximus*, fem. *maxima*, neut. *maximum*).
- **Meatus**, pl. **meatus**, gen. **meatus**. Meatus, canal. 4th declension masc.
- **Medialis**, pl. **mediales**, gen. **medialis**. Medial. 3rd declension masc./fem. (adj.: masc. *medialis*, fem. *medialis*, neut. *mediale*)
- **Medium**, pl. **media**, gen. **medii**. Substance, culture medium, means. 2nd declension neut.
- **Medulla**, pl. **medullae**, gen. **medullae**. Marrow. 1st declension fem.
  - *Medulla oblongata* (caudal portion of the brainstem), *medulla spinalis*
- **Membrana**, pl. **membranae**, gen. **membranae**. Membrane. 1st declension fem.
- **Membrum**, pl. **membra**, gen. **membri**. Limb. 2nd declension neut.
- **Meningitis**, pl. **meningitides**, gen. **meningitidis**. Meningitis. 3rd declension fem.
- **Meningococcus**, pl. **meningococci**, gen. **meningococci**. Meningococcus. 2nd declension masc.
- **Meninx**, pl. **meninges**, gen. **meningis**. Meninx. 3rd declension.
- **Meniscus**, pl. **menisci**, gen. **menisci**. Meniscus. 2nd declension masc.
- **Mentum**, pl. **menti**, gen. **menti**. Chin. 2nd declension masc.
- **Mesocardium**, pl. **mesocardia**, gen. **mesocardii**. Mesocardium. 2nd declension neut.
- **Mesothelium**, pl. **mesothelia**, gen. **mesothelii**. Mesothelium. 2nd declension neut.
- **Metacarpus**, pl. **metacarpi**, gen. **metacarpi**. Metacarpus. 2nd declension masc.
- **Metaphysis**, pl. **metaphyses**, gen. **metaphysis**. Metaphysis. 3rd declension.
- **Metastasis**, pl. **metastases**, gen. **metastasis**. Metastasis. 3rd declension
- **Metatarsus**, pl. **metatarsi**, gen. **metatarsi**. Metatarsus. 2nd declension masc.
- **Microvillus**, pl. **microvilli**, gen. **microvilli**. Microvillus (from *villus*, hair). 2nd declension masc.
- **Minimus**, pl. **minimi**, gen. **minimi**. The smallest, the least. 2nd declension masc. (adj,: masc. *minimus*, fem. *minima*, neut. *minimum*).
- **Minor**, pl. **minores**, gen. **minoris**. Lesser. 3rd declension masc.
- **Mitochondrion**, pl. **mitochondria**, gen. **mitochondrium**. Mitochondrion. 3rd declension neut.
- **Mitosis**, pl. **mitoses**, gen. **mitosis**. Mitosis. 3rd declension (from Gr. *mitos*, thread).
- **Mons**, pl. **montes**, gen. **montis**. Mons (lit. *mountain*). 3rd declension masc.
- **Mors**, pl. **mortes**, gen. **mortis**, acc. **mortem**. Death. 3rd declension fem.
- **Mucolipidosis**, pl. **mucolipidoses**, gen. **mucolipidosis**. Mucolipidosis. 3rd declension masc./fem.

- **Mucro, pl. mucrones, gen. mucronis.** Sharp-tipped structure. 3rd declension masc.
  - *Mucro sterni* (sternal xyphoides).
- **Musculus, pl. musculi, gen. musculi.** Muscle. 2nd declension masc.
- **Mycelium, pl. mycelia, gen. mycelii.** Mycelium, mass of hyphae. 2nd declension neut.
- **Mycoplasma, pl. mycoplasmata, gen. mycoplasmatis.** Mycoplasma. 3rd declension neut.
- **Mylohyoideus m., pl. mylohyoidei, gen. mylohyoidei.** 2nd declension masc.
- **Myocardium, pl. myocardia, gen. myocardii.** Myocardium. 2nd declension neut.
- **Myofibrilla, pl. myofibrillae, gen. myofibrillae.** Myofibrilla. 1st declension fem.
- **Myrinx, pl. myringes, gen. myringis.** Eardrum. 3rd declension.

N

- **Naris, pl. nares, gen. naris.** Nostril. 3rd declension fem.
- **Nasus, pl. nasi, gen. nasi.** Nose. 2nd declension masc.
- **Navicularis, pl. naviculares, gen. navicularis.** Ship shaped. 3rd declension masc.
- **Nebula, pl. nebulae, gen. nebulae.** Mist, cloud (corneal nebula. corneal opacity). 1st declension fem.
- **Neisseria, pl. neisseriae, gen. neisseriae.** Neisseria. 1st declension fem.
- **Nephritis, pl. nephritides, gen. nephritidis.** Nephritis. 3rd declension.
- **Nervus, pl. nervi, gen. nervi.** Nerve. 2nd declension masc.
- **Neuritis, pl. neuritides, gen. neuritidis.** Neuritis. 3rd declension.
- **Neurosis, pl. neuroses, gen. neurosis.** Neurosis. 3rd declension.
- **Nevus, pl. nevi, gen. nevi.** Nevus (lit. mole on the body, birthmark). 2nd declension masc.
- **Nidus, pl. nidi, gen. nidi.** Nidus (lit. *nest*). 2nd declension masc.
- **Nodulus, pl. noduli, gen. noduli.** Nodule (small node, knot). 2nd declension masc.
- **Nucleolus, pl. nucleoli, gen. nucleoli.** Nucleolus (small nucleus). 2nd declension masc.
- **Nucleus, pl. nuclei, gen. nuclei.** Nucleus (central part, core, lit. *inside of a nut*). 2nd declension masc.

O

- **Obliquus, pl. obliqui, gen. obliqui.** Oblique. 2nd declension masc. (adj.: masc. *obliquus*, fem. *obliqua*, neut. *obliquum*).
- **Occiput, pl. occipita, gen. occipitis.** Occiput (back of the head). 3rd declension neut.
- **Oculentum, pl. oculenta, gen. oculenti.** Eye ointment. 2nd declension neut.
- **Oculus, pl. oculi, gen. oculi.** Eye. 2nd declension masc.

- **Oliva, pl. olivae, gen. olivae.** Rounded elevation (lit. *olive*). 1st declension fem.
- **Omentum, pl. omenta, gen. omenti.** Peritoneal fold. 2nd declension neut.
- **Oogonium, pl. oogonia, gen. oogonii.** Oocyte. 2nd declension neut.
- **Operculum, pl. opercula, gen. operculi.** Operculum, cover (lit. *lesser lid*). 2nd declension neut.
- **Orbicularis m., pl. orbiculares, gen. orbicularis.** Muscle encircling a structure. 3rd declension masc. (adj.: masc. *orbicularis*, fem. *orbicularis*, neut. *orbiculare*).
- **Organum, pl. organa, gen. organi.** Organ. 2nd declension neuter.
- **Orificium, pl. orificia, gen. orificii.** Opening, orifice. 2nd declension neuter.
- **Os, pl. ora, gen. oris.** Mouth. 3rd declension neut.
- **Os, pl. ossa, gen. ossis.** Bone. 3rd declension neut.
  - *Os* + genitive case: *os coccyges* (coccigeal bone), *os ischii* (ischium).
- **Ossiculum, pl. ossicula, gen. ossiculi.** Ossicle, small bone. 2nd declension masc.
- **Ostium, pl. ostia, gen. ostii.** Opening into a tubular organ, entrance. 2nd declension neuter.
- **Ovalis, pl. ovales, gen. ovalis.** Oval. 3rd declension masc. (adj.: masc. *ovalis*, fem. *ovalis*, neut. *ovale*)
- **Ovarium, pl. ovaria, gen. ovarii.** Ovary. 2nd declension neut.
- **Ovulum, pl. ovula, gen. ovuli.** Ovule. 2nd declension neut.

P

- **Palatum, pl. palata, gen. palati.** Palate. 2nd declension neut.
- **Palma, pl. palmae, gen. palmae.** Palm. 1st declension fem.
- **Palmaris, pl. palmares, gen. palmaris.** Relative to the palm of the hand. 3rd declension masc. (adj.: masc. *palmaris*, fem. *palmaris*, neut. *palmare*).
- **Palpebra, pl. palpebrae, gen. palpebrae.** Eyelid. 1st declension fem.
- **Pancreas, pl. pancreates/pancreata, gen. pancreatis.** Pancreas. 3rd declension fem./neut.
- **Panniculus, pl. panniculi, gen. panniculi.** Panniculus (a layer of tissue, from *pannus*, pl. *panni*, cloth). 2nd declension masc.
- **Pannus, pl. panni, gen. panni.** Pannus (lit. *cloth*). 2nd declension masc.
- **Papilla, pl. papillae, gen. papillae.** Papilla (lit. *nipple*). 1st declension fem.
- **Paralysis, pl. paralyses, gen. paralysos/paralysis.** Palsy. 3rd declension fem.
- **Parametrium, pl. parametria, gen. parametrii.** Parametrium. 2nd declension neut.
- **Paries, pl. parietes, gen. parietis.** Wall. 3rd declension masc.
- **Pars, pl. partes, gen. partis.** Part. 3rd declension fem.
- **Patella, pl. patellae, gen. patellae.** Patella. 1st declension fem.
- **Pectoralis m., pl. pectorales, gen. pectoralis.** Pectoralis muscle. 3rd declension masc. (adj.: masc. *pectoralis*, fem. *pectoralis*, neut. *pectorale*).

- **Pectus**, pl. **pectora**, gen. **pectoris**. Chest. 3rd declension neut.
  - *Pectus excavatum, pectus carinatum.*
- **Pediculus**, pl. **pediculi**, gen. **pediculi**. 1. Pedicle. 2. Louse. 2nd declension masc.
- **Pedunculus**, pl. **pedunculi**, gen. **pedunculi**. Pedicle. 2nd declension masc.
- **Pelvis**, pl. **pelves**, gen. **pelvis**. Pelvis. 3rd declension fem.
- **Penis**, pl. **penes**, gen. **penis**. Penis. 3rd declension masc.
- **Perforans**, pl. **perforantes**, gen. **perforantis**. Something which pierces a structure. 3rd declension masc.
- **Pericardium**, pl. **pericardia**, gen. **pericardii**. Pericardium. 2nd declension neut.
- **Perimysium**, pl. **perimysia**, gen. **perimysii**. Perimysium (from Gr. *mysia*, muscle). 2nd declension neut.
- **Perineum**, pl. **perinea**, gen. **perinei**. Perineum. 2nd declension neut.
- **Perineurium**, pl. **perineuria**, gen. **perineurii**. Perineurium (from Gr. *neuron*, nerve). 2nd declension neut.
- **Periodontium**, pl. **periodontia**, gen. **periodontii**. Periodontium (from Gr. *odous*, tooth). 2nd declension neut.
- **Perionychium**, pl. **perionychia**, gen. **perionychii**. Perionychium (from Gr. *onyx*, nail). 2nd declension neut.
- **Periosteum**, pl. **periostea**, gen. **periosteii**. Periosteum (from Gr. *osteon*, bone). 2nd declension neut.
- **Periostosis**, pl. **periostoses**, gen. **periostosis**. Periostosis. 3rd declension.
- **Peritoneum**, pl. **peritonea**, gen. **peritonei**. Peritoneum. 2nd declension neut.
- **Peroneus m.**, pl. **peronei**, gen. **peronei**. Peroneal bone. 2nd declension masc.
- **Pes**, pl. **pedes**, gen. **pedis**. Foot. 3rd declension masc.
- **Petechia**, pl. **petechiae**, gen. **petechiae**. Petechiae (tiny hemorrhagic spots). 1st declension fem.
- **Phalanx**, pl. **phalanges**, gen. **phalangis**. Phalanx (long bones of the digits). 3rd declension fem.
  - *Os phalangi*, pl. *ossa phalangium.*
- **Phallus**, pl. **phalli**, gen. **phalli**. Penis. 2nd declension masc.
- **Pharynx**, pl. **pharynges**, gen. **pharyngis**. Pharynx. 3rd declension.
- **Philtrum**, pl. **philtra**, gen. **philtri**. Philtrum. 2nd declension neut.
- **Phimosis**, pl. **phimoses**, gen. **phimosis**. Phimosis. 3rd declension masc.
- **Phlyctena**, pl. **phlyctenae**, gen. **phlyctenae**. Phlyctena (small blister). 1st declension fem.
- **Pia mater**, pl. **piae matres**, gen. **piae matris**. Pia mater (inner meningeal layer of tissue). 1st declension fem. (adj.: masc. *pius*, fem. *pia*, neut. *pium*, tender).
- **Placenta**, pl. **placentae**, gen. **placentae**. Placenta (lit. *cake*). 1st declension fem.
- **Planta**, pl. **plantae**, gen. **plantae**. Plant, sole. 1st declension fem.

- **Plantar**, pl. **plantaria**, gen. **plantaris**. Relating to the sole of the foot. 3rd declension neut.
- **Planum**, pl. **plana**, gen. **plani**. Plane. 2nd declension neut.
- **Platysma m.**, pl. **platysmata**, gen. **platysmatis**. Platysma. 3rd declension neut.
- **Pleura**, pl. **pleurae**, gen. **pleurae**. Pleura. 1st declension fem.
- **Plica**, pl. **plicae**, gen. **plicae**. Fold. 1st declension fem.
- **Pneumoconiosis**, pl. **pneumoconioses**, gen. **pneumoconiosis**. Pneumoconiosis. 3rd declension.
- **Pollex**, pl. **pollices**, gen. **pollicis**. Thumb. 3rd declension masc.
- **Polus**, pl. **poli**, gen. **poli**. Pole. 2nd declension masc.
- **Pons**, pl. **pontes**, gen. **pontis**. Pons (lit. *bridge*). 3rd declension masc.
- **Porta**, pl. **portae**, gen. **portae**. Porta (from Lat. verb *porto*, carry, bring). 1st declension fem.
- **Portio**, pl. **portiones**, gen. **portionis**. Portion. 3rd declension fem.
- **Porus**, pl. **pori**, gen. **pori**. Pore. 2nd declension masc.
- **Posterior**, pl. **posteriores**, gen. **posterioris**. Coming after. 3rd declension.
- **Praeputium**, pl. **praeputia**, gen. **praeputii**. Prepuce, foreskin. 2nd declension neut.
- **Princeps**, pl. **principes**, gen. **principis**. First, foremost, leading. 3rd declension masc.
- **Processus**, pl. **processus**, gen. **processus**. Process. 4th declension masc.
- **Profunda**, pl. **profundae**, gen. **profundae**. Deep. 1st declension fem. (adj.: masc. *profundus*, fem. *profunda*, neut. *profundum*).
  - *Vena femoralis profunda*, deep femoral vein.
- **Prominentia**, pl. **prominentiae**, gen. **prominentiae**. Prominence. 1st declension fem.
- **Promontorium**, pl. **promontoria**, gen. **promontorii**. Promontorium. 2nd declension neut.
- **Pronator**, pl. **pronatores**, gen. **pronatoris**. A muscle that serves to pronate. 3rd declension masc.
  - *Pronator teres m., pronator quadratus m.*
- **Prophylaxis**, pl. **prophylaxes**, gen. **prophylaxis**. Prophylaxis (from Gr. *prophylasso*, take precaution). 3rd declension.
- **Proprius**, pl. **proprii**, gen. **proprii**. Own. 2nd declension masc. (adj.: masc. *proprius*, fem. *propria*, neut. *proprium*)
- **Prosthesis**, pl. **prostheses**, gen. **prosthesis**. Prosthesis. 3rd declension fem.
- **Psychosis**, pl. **psychoses**, gen. **psychosis**. Psychosis. 3rd declension fem.
- **Ptosis**, pl. **ptoses**, gen. **ptosis**. Ptosis. 3rd declension.
- **Pubes**, pl. **pubes**, gen. **pubis**. Pubis. 3rd declension fem.
- **Pudendum**, pl. **pudenda**, gen. **pudendi**. Relative to the external genitals (lit. *shameful*). 2nd declension neut. (adj.: masc. *pudendus*, fem. *pudenda*, neut. *pudendum*).
- **Puerpera**, pl. **puerperae**, gen. **puerperae**. Puerpera. 1st declension fem.
- **Puerperium**, pl. **puerperia**, gen. **puerperii**. Puerperium. 2nd declension neut.

- **Pulmo**, pl. **pulmones**, gen. **pulmonis**. Lung. 3rd declension masc.
- **Punctata**, pl. **punctatae**, gen. **puctatae**. Pointed. 1st declension fem.
- **Punctum**, pl. **puncta**, gen. **puncti**. Point. 2nd declension neut.
- **Pylorus**, pl. **pylori**, gen. **pylori**. Pylorus. 2nd declension masc.
- **Pyramidalis m.**, pl. **pyramidales**, gen. **pyramidalis**. Pyramidal. 3rd declension masc. (adj.: masc. *pyramidalis*, fem. *pyramidalis*, neut. *pyramidale*).
- **Pyriformis m.**, pl. **pyriformes**, gen. **pyriformis**. Pear-shaped. 3rd declension masc. (adj.: masc. *pyriformis*, fem. *pyriformis*, neut. *pyriforme*).

Q

- **Quadratus**, pl. **quadrati**, gen. **quadrati**. Square. 2nd declension masc. (adj.: masc. *quadratus*, fem. *quadrata*, neut. *quadratum*).
- **Quadrigemina**, pl. **quadrigeminae**, gen. **quadrigeminae**. Fourfold, in four parts. 1st declension fem. (adj.: *quadrigeminus*, fem. *quadrigemina*, neut. *quadrigeminum*)

R

- **Rachis**, pl. Lat. **rachides**, pl. Engl. **rachises**, gen. **rachidis**. Rachis, vertebral column. 3rd declension.
- **Radiatio**, pl. **radiationes**, gen. **radiationis**. Radiation. 3rd declension fem.
- **Radius**, pl. **radii**, gen. **radii**. Radius. 2nd declension masc.
- **Radix**, pl. **radices**, gen. **radicis**. Root, base. 3rd declension fem.
- **Ramus**, pl. **rami**, gen. **rami**. Branch. 2nd declension masc.
- **Receptaculum**, pl. **receptacula**, gen. **receptaculi**. Receptacle, reservoir. 2nd declension neut.
- **Recessus**, pl. **recessus**, gen. **recessus**. Recess. 4th declension masc.
- **Rectus**, pl. **recti**, gen. **recti**. Right, straight (adj.: masc. *rectus*, fem. *recta*, neut. *rectum*).
  - *Rectus abdominis m.*
- **Regio**, pl. **regiones**, gen. **regionis**. Region. 3rd declension fem.
- **Ren**, pl. **renes**, gen. **renis**. Kidney. 3rd declension masc.
- **Rete**, pl. **retia**, gen. **retis**. Network, net. 3rd declension neut.
  - *Rete mirabilis.*
- **Reticulum**, pl. **reticula**, gen. **reticuli**. Reticulum. 2nd declension neut.
- **Retinaculum**, pl. **retinacula**, gen. **retinaculi**. Retinaculum (retaining band or ligament). 2nd declension neut.
- **Rima**, pl. **rimae**, gen. **rima**. Fissure, slit. 1st declension fem.
- **Rostrum**, pl. **rostra**, gen. **rostri**. Rostrum (beak-shaped structure). 2nd declension neut.
- **Rotundum**, pl. **rotunda**, gen. **rotundi**. Round declension (adj.: masc. *rotundus*, fem. *rotunda*, neut. *rotundum*).
  - *Foramen rotundum*, pl. *foramina rotunda.*
- **Ruga**, pl. **rugae**, gen. **rugae**. Wrinkle, fold. 1st declension fem.

S

- Sacculus, pl. **sacculi**, gen. **sacculi**. Small pouch. 2nd declension masc.
- Saccus, pl. **sacci**, gen. **sacci**. Pouch. 2nd declension masc.
- Sacrum, pl. **sacra**, gen. **sacri**. Sacral bone (lit. *sacred vessel*). 2nd declension neut.
- Salpinx, pl. **salpinges**, gen. **salpingis**. Fallopian tube. 3rd declension.
- Sartorius m., pl. **sartorii**, gen. **sartorii**. Sartorius muscle (tailor's muscle). 2nd declension masc.
- Scalenus m., gen. **scaleni**, pl. **scaleni**. Uneven. 2nd declension masc.
- Scapula, pl. **scapulae**, gen. **scapulae**. Scapula, shoulder blade. 1st declension fem.
- Sclerosis, pl. **scleroses**, gen. **sclerosis**. Sclerosis . 3rd declension.
- Scolex, pl. **scoleces**, gen. **scolecis**. Scolex. 3rd declension.
- Scotoma, pl. **scotomata**, gen. **scotomatis**. Scotoma. 3rd declension neut.
- Scrotum, pl. **scrota**, gen. **scroti**. Scrotum. 2nd declension neut.
- Scutulum, pl. **scutula**, gen. **scutuli**. Scutulum. 2nd declension neut.
- Scybalum, pl. **scybala**, gen. **scybali**. Scybalum. 2nd declension neut.
- Segmentum, pl. **segmenta**, gen. **segmenti**. Segment. 2nd declension neut.
- Sella turcica, pl. **sellae turcicae**, gen. **sellae turcicae**. Turkish chair. 1st declension fem.
- Semen, pl. **semina**, gen. **seminis**. Semen. 3rd declension neut.
- Semimembranosus m., pl. **semimembranosi**, gen. **semimembranosi**. 2nd declension masc.
- Semitendinosus m., pl. **semitendinosi**, gen. **semitendinosi**. 2nd declension masc.
- Sensorium, pl. **sensoria**, gen. **sensorii**. Sensorium. 2nd declension neut.
- Sepsis, pl. **sepses**, gen. **sepsis**. Sepsis. 3rd declension.
- Septum, pl. **septa**, gen. **septi**. Septum. 2nd declension neut.
- Sequela, pl. **sequelae**, gen. **sequelae**. Sequela. 1st declension fem.
- Sequestrum, pl. **sequestra**, gen. **sequestri**. Sequestrum (from sequester, go-between). 2nd declension neut.
- Serosa, pl. **serosae**, gen. **serosae**. Serosa. 1st declension fem.
- Serratus m., pl. **serrati**, gen. **serrati**. Serrated, toothed like a saw. 2nd declension masc.
- Serum, pl. **sera**, gen. **seri**. Serum (lit. *whey*). 2nd declension neut.
- Sinciput, pl. **sincipita**, gen. **sincipitis**. Sinciput. 3rd declension neut.
- Sinus, pl. **sinus**, gen. **sinus**. Sinus. 4th declension masc.
- Soleus m., pl. **solei**, gen. **solei**. Soleus. 2nd declension masc.
- Spatium, pl. **spatia**, gen. **spatii**. Space. 2nd declension neut.
- Spectrum, pl. **spectra**, gen. **spectri**. Spectrum. 2nd declension neut.
- Sphincter, pl. Lat. **sphincteres**, pl. Engl. **sphincters**, gen. **sphincteris**. Sphincter. 3rd declension masc.
- Spiculum, pl. **spicula**, gen. **spiculi**. Spike (lit. *sting*). 2nd declension neut.
- Spina, pl. **spinae**, gen. **spinae**. Spine. 1st declension fem.
- Splenium, pl. **splenia**, gen. **splenii**. Splenium. 2nd declension neut.
  - *Splenius capitis/colli mm.*

- **Splenunculus**, pl. **splenunculi**, gen. **splenunculi**. Accessory spleen. 2nd declension masc.
- **Sputum**, pl. **sputa**, gen. **sputi**. Sputum. 2nd declension neut.
- **Squama**, pl. **squamae**, gen. **squamae**. Squama (scale, plate-like structure). 1st declension fem.
- **Stapes**, pl. **stapedes**, gen. **stapedis**. Stapes. 3rd declension masc.
- **Staphylococcus**, pl. **staphylococci**, gen. **staphylococci**. Staphylococcus. 2nd declension masc.
- **Stasis**, pl. **stases**, gen. **stasis**. Stasis. 3rd declension masc.
- **Statoconium**, pl. **statoconia**, gen. **statoconii**. Statoconium. 2nd declension neut.
- **Stenosis**, pl. **stenoses**, gen. **stenosis**. Stenosis. 3rd declension.
- **Stereocilium**, pl. **stereocilia**, gen. **stereocilii**. Stereocilium. 2nd declension neut.
- **Sternocleidomastoideus m.**, pl. **sternocleidomastoidei**, gen. **sternocleidomastoidei**. 2nd declension masc.
- **Sternum**, pl. **sterna**, gen. **sterni**. Sternum. 2nd declension neut.
- **Stigma**, pl. **stigmata**, gen. **stigmatis**. Stigma (mark aiding in diagnosis). 3rd declension neut.
- **Stimulus**, pl. **stimuli**, gen. **stimuli**. Stimulus (lit. *spur*). 2nd declension masc.
- **Stoma**, pl. **stomata**, gen. **stomatis**. Stoma, opening, hole. 3rd declension neut.
- **Stratum**, pl. **strata**, gen. **strati**. Stratum. 2nd declension neut.
- **Stria**, pl. **striae**, gen. **striae**. Fluting, channel. 1st declension fem.
- **Stroma**, pl. **stromata**, gen. **stromatis**. Stroma. 3rd declension neut.
- **Struma**, pl. **strumae**, gen. **strumae**. Struma. 1st declension fem.
- **Subiculum**, pl. **subicula**, gen. **subiculi**. Subiculum. 2nd declension neut.
- **Substantia**, pl. **substantiae**, gen. **substantiae**. Substance. 1st declension fem.
- **Sulcus**, pl. **sulci**, gen. **sulci**. Sulcus (lit. furrow, wrinkle). 2nd declension masc.
- **Supercilium**, pl. **supercilia**, gen. **supercilii**. Eyebrow. 2nd declension neut.
- **Superficialis**, pl. **superficiales**, gen. **superficialis**. Superficial. 3rd declension masc. (adj.: masc. *superficialis*, fem. *superficialis*, neut. *superficiale*).
- **Superior**, pl. **superiores**, gen. **superioris**. Higher, upper, greater. 3rd declension.
- **Sustentaculum**, pl. **sustentacula**, gen. **sustentaculi**. Sustentaculum. 2nd declension neut.
- **Sutura**, pl. **suturae**, gen. **suturae**. Suture. 1st declension fem.
- **Symphysis**, pl. **symphyses**, gen. **symphysis**. Symphysis. 3rd declension.
- **Synchondrosis**, pl. **synchondroses**, gen. **synchondrosis**. Synchondrosis. 3rd declension.
- **Syncytium**, pl. **syncytia**, gen. **syncytii**. Syncytium. 2nd declension neut.

- **Syndesmosis**, pl. **syndesmoses**, gen. **syndesmosis**. Syndesmosis. 3rd declension.
- **Synechia**, pl. **synechiae**, gen. **synechiae**. Synechia. 1st declension fem.
- **Syrinx**, pl. **syringes**, gen. **syringis**. Syrinx. 3rd declension.

T

- **Talus**, pl. **tali**, gen. **tali**. Talus. 2nd declension masc.
- **Tarsus**, pl. **tarsi**, gen. **tarsi**. Tarsus. 2nd declension masc.
- **Tectum**, pl. **tecta**, gen. **tecti**. Roof. 2nd declension neut.
- **Tegmen**, pl. **tegmina**, gen. **tegminis**. Roof, covering. 3rd declension neut.
- **Tegmentum**, pl. **tegmenta**, gen. **tegmenti**. Covering. 2nd declension neut.
- **Tela**, pl. **telae**, gen. **telae**. Membrane (lit. *web*). 1st declension fem.
- **Telangiectasis**, pl. **telangiectases**, gen. **telangiectasis**. Telangiectasis. 3rd declension.
- **Temporalis m.**, pl. **temporales**, gen. **temporalis**. 3rd declension masc. (adj.: masc. *temporalis*, fem. *temporalis*, neut. *temporale*).
- **Tenaculum**, pl. **tenacula**, gen. **tenaculi**. Surgical clamp. 2nd declension neut.
- **Tendo**, pl. **tendines**, gen. **tendinis**. Tendon, sinew (from verb *tendo*, stretch). 3rd.
- **Tenia**, pl. **teniae**, gen. **teniae**. Tenia. 1st declension fem.
- **Tensor**, pl. **tensores**, gen. **tensoris**. Something that stretches, that tenses a muscle. 3rd declension masc.
- **Tentorium**, pl. **tentoria**, gen. **tentorii**. Tentorium. 2nd declension neut.
- **Teres**, pl. **teretes**, gen. **teretis**. Round and long. 3rd declension masc.
- **Testis**, pl. **testes**, gen. **testis**. Testicle. 3rd declension masc.
- **Thalamus**, pl. **thalami**, gen. **thalami**. Thalamus (lit. *marriage bed*). 2nd declension masc.
- **Theca**, pl. **thecae**, gen. **thecae**. Theca, envelope (lit. *case, box*). 1st declension fem.
- **Thelium**, pl. **thelia**, gen. **thelii**. Nipple. 2nd declension neut.
- **Thenar**, pl. **thenares**, gen. **thenaris**. Relative to the palm of the hand. 3rd declension neut.
- **Thesis**, pl. **theses**, gen. **thesis**. Thesis. 3rd declension fem.
- **Thorax**, pl. **thoraces**, gen. **thoracos/thoracis**. Chest. 3rd declension masc.
- **Thrombosis**, pl. **thromboses**, gen. **thombosis**. Thrombosis. 3rd declension.
- **Thrombus**, pl. **thrombi**, gen. **thrombi**. Thrombus, clot (from Gr. *thrombos*). 2nd declension masc.
- **Thymus**, pl. **thymi**, gen. **thymi**. Thymus. 2nd declension masc.
- **Tibia**, pl. **tibiae**, gen. **tibiae**. Tibia. 1st declension fem.
- **Tonsilla**, pl. **tonsillae**, gen. **tonsillae**. Tonsil. 1st declension fem.
- **Tophus**, pl. **tophi**, gen. **tophi**. Tophus. 2nd declension masc.
- **Torulus**, pl. **toruli**, gen. **toruli**. Papilla, small elevation. 2nd declension masc.
- **Trabecula**, pl. **trabeculae**, gen. **trabeculae**. Trabecula (supporting bundle of either osseous or fibrous fibers). 1st declension fem.

- **Trachea**, pl. **tracheae**, gen. **tracheae**. Trachea. 1st declension fem.
- **Tractus**, pl. **tractus**, gen. **tractus**. Tract. 4th declension masc.
- **Tragus**, pl. **tragi**, gen. **tragi**. Tragus, hircus. 2nd declension masc.
- **Transversalis**, pl. **transversales**, gen. **transversalis**. Transverse. 3rd declension. (adj.: masc. *transversalis*, fem. *transversalis*, neut. *transversale*).
- **Transversus**, pl. **transversi**, gen. **transversi**. Lying across, from side to side. 2nd declension masc. (adj.: masc. *transversus*, fem. *transversa*, neut. *transversum*).
- **Trapezium**, pl. **trapezia**, gen. **trapezii**. Trapezium bone. 2nd declension neut.
- **Trauma**, pl. **traumata**, gen. **traumatis**. Trauma. 3rd declension neut.
- **Triangularis**, pl. **triangulares**, gen. **triangularis**. Triangular. 3rd declension masc. (adj.: masc. *triangularis*, fem. *triangularis*, neut. *triangulare*).
- **Triceps**, pl. **tricipes**, gen. **tricipis**. Triceps (from *ceps*, pl. *cipes*, gen. *cipis*, headed). 3rd declension masc.
- **Trigonum**, pl. **trigona**, gen. **trigoni**. Trigonum (lit. *triangle*). 2nd declension neut.
- **Triquetrum**, pl. **triquetra**, gen. **triquetri**. Triquetrum, triquetral bone, pyramidal bone. 2nd declension neut. (adj.: masc. *triquetrus*, fem. *triquetra*, neut. *triquetrum*. Three-cornered, triangular).
- **Trochlea**, pl. **trochleae**, gen. **trochleae**. Trochlea (lit. *pulley*). 1st declension fem.
- **Truncus**, pl. **trunci**, gen. **trunci**. Trunk. 2nd declension masc.
- **Tuba**, pl. **tubae**, gen. **tubae**. Tube. 1st declension fem.
- **Tuberculum**, pl. **tubercula**, gen. **tuberculi**. Tuberculum, swelling, protuberance. 2nd declension neut.
- **Tubulus**, pl. **tubuli**, gen. **tubuli**. Tubule. 2nd declension masc.
- **Tunica**, pl. **tunicae**, gen. **tunicae**. Tunic. 1st declension fem.
- **Tylosis**, pl. **tyloses**, gen. **tylosis**. Tylosis (callosity). 3rd declension.
- **Tympanum**, pl. **tympana**, gen. **tympani**. Tympanum, eardrum (lit. *small drum*). 2nd declension neut.

U

- **Ulcus**, pl. **ulcera**, gen. **ulceris**. Ulcer. 3rd declension neut.
- **Ulna**, pl. **ulnae**, gen. **ulnae**. Ulna (lit. *forearm*). 1st declension fem.
- **Umbilicus**, pl. **umbilici**, gen. **umbiculi**. Navel. 2nd declension masc.
- **Uncus**, pl. **unci**, gen. **unci**. Uncus (lit. *hook*, *clamp*). 2nd declension masc.
- **Unguis**, pl. **ungues**, gen. **unguis**. Nail, claw. 3rd declension masc.
- **Uterus**, pl. **uteri**, gen. **uteri**. Uterus, womb. 2nd declension masc.
- **Utriculus**, pl. **utriculi**, gen. **utriculi**. Utriculus (lit. *wineskin*). 2nd declension masc.
- **Uveitis**, pl. **uveitides**, gen. **uveitidis**. Uveitis. 3rd declension fem.
- **Uvula**, pl. **uvulae**, gen. **uvulae**. Uvula (lit. *small grape*, from *uva*, pl. *uvae*, grape). 1st declension fem.

V

- **Vagina,** pl. **vaginae,** gen. **vaginae.** Vagina, sheath. 1st declension fem.
- **Vaginitis,** pl. **vaginitides,** gen. **vaginitidis.** Vaginitis. 3rd declension fem.
- **Vagus,** pl. **vagi,** gen. **vagi.** Vagus nerve. 2nd declension masc. (adj.: masc. *vagus,* fem. *vaga,* neut. *vagum.* Roving, wandering).
- **Valva,** pl. **valvae,** gen. **valvae.** Leaflet. 1st declension fem.
- **Valvula,** pl. **valvulae,** gen. **valvulae.** Valve. 1st declension fem.
- **Varix,** pl. **varices,** gen. **varicis.** Varix, varicose vein. 3rd declension masc.
- **Vas,** pl. **vasa,** gen. **vasis.** Vessel. 3rd declension neut.
  - *Vas deferens, vasa recta, vasa vasorum.*
- **Vasculum,** pl. **vascula,** gen. **vasculi.** Small vessel. 2nd declension neut.
- **Vastus,** pl. **vasti,** gen. **vasti.** Vast, huge. 2nd declension neut. (adj.: masc. *vastus,* fem. *vasta,* neut. *vasti*).
  - *Vastus medialis/intermedius/lateralis m.*
- **Vasum,** pl. **vasa,** gen. **vasi.** Vessel. 2nd declension neut.
- **Velum,** pl. **veli,** gen. **veli.** Covering, curtain (lit. *sail*). 2nd declension neut.
- **Vena,** pl. **venae,** gen. **venae.** Vein. 1st declension fem.
  - *Vena cava,* pl. *venae cavae,* gen. *venae cavae* (from masc. cavus, fem. cava, neut. cavum, hollow).
- **Ventriculus,** pl. **ventriculi,** gen. **ventriculi.** Ventricle (lit. *small belly*). 2nd declension masc.
- **Venula,** pl. **venulae,** gen. **venulae.** Venule. 1st declension fem.
- **Vermis,** pl. **vermes,** gen. **vermis.** Worm. 3rd declension masc.
- **Verruca,** pl. **verrucae,** gen. **verrucae.** Wart. 1st declension fem.
- **Vertebra,** pl. **vertebrae,** gen. **vertebrae.** Vertebra. 1st declension fem.
- **Vertex,** pl. **vertices,** gen. **verticis.** Vertex (lit. *peak, top*). 3rd declension masc.
- **Vesica,** pl. **vesicae,** gen. **vesicae.** Bladder. 1st declension fem.
- **Vesicula,** pl. **vesiculae,** gen. **vesiculae.** Vesicle (lit. *lesser bladder*). 1st declension fem.
- **Vestibulum,** pl. **vestibula,** gen. **vestibuli.** Entrance to a cavity. 2nd declension neut.
- **Villus,** pl. **villi,** gen. **villi.** Villus (shaggy hair). 2nd declension masc.
- **Vinculum,** pl. **vincula,** gen. **vinculi.** Band, band-like structure (lit. *chain, bond*). 2nd declension neut.
- **Virus,** pl. Lat. **viri,** pl. Engl. **viruses,** gen. **viri.** Virus. 2nd declension masc.
- **Viscus,** pl. **viscera,** gen. **visceris.** Viscus, internal organ. 3rd declension neut.
- **Vitiligo,** pl. **vitiligines,** gen. **vitiligis.** Vitiligo. 3rd declension masc.
- **Vomer,** pl. **vomeres,** gen. **vomeris.** Vomer bone. 3rd declension masc.
- **Vulva,** pl. **vulvae,** gen. **vulvae.** Vulva. 1st declension fem.

Z

- **Zona**, pl. **zonae**, gen. **zonae**. Zone. 1st declension fem.
- **Zonula**, pl. **zonulae**, gen. **zonulae**. Small zone. 1st declension fem.
- **Zygapophysis**, pl. **zygapophyses**, gen. **zygapophysis**. Vertebral articular apophysis. 3rd declension fem.

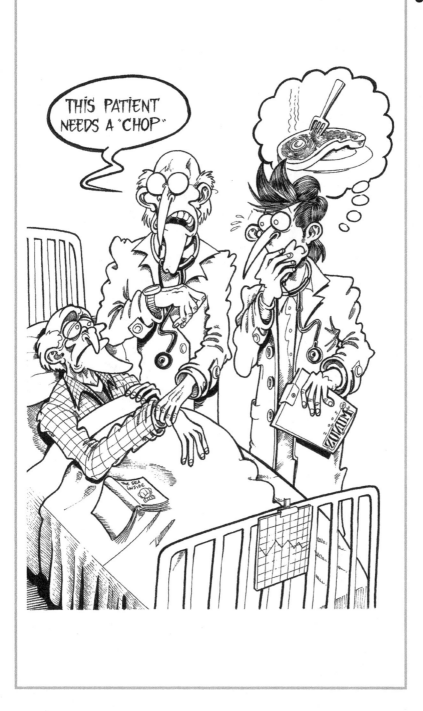

Unit X   Acronyms and Abbreviations

Introduction

"The patient went from the ER to the OR and then to the ICU."

It is an irrefutable fact that doctors' speech is full of abbreviations. Health-care professionals in general and radiologists in particular use at least ten abbreviations per minute (this is our own home-made statistic; please don't quote us). This high prevalence has led us to consider medical abbreviations as a challenging pandemic.

There are several "types" of abbreviations, namely:

- Straightforward abbreviations
- Extra-nice abbreviations
- Expanded-term abbreviations
- Energy-saving abbreviations
- Double-meaning abbreviations
- Mind-blowing abbreviations

Let us begin with the nice ones; we call them the *straightforward* abbreviations because for each nice abbreviation in your own language there is a nice English equivalent. No beating around the bush here. It's just a matter of changing letter order, identifying the abbreviations and learning them. Let us give you a few examples so you can enjoy the simple things in life ... while you can!

HRT   Hormone replacement therapy
LVOT   Left ventricle outflow tract
ASD   Atrial septal defect
VSD   Ventricular septal defect
TEE   Transesophageal echocardiography
LDA   Left anterior descending artery
ACE   Angiotensin converting enzyme

There are other kinds of abbreviation: the *extra-nice* ones. They are mostly used for drugs or chemical substances whose name has three or four syllables too many. They are extra nice because they are usually the same in many languages. Let's see just an example:

CPK   Creatine phosphokinase

In the next group, we have put together some examples of abbreviations that are widely used in English but that are generally preferred in their expanded form in other languages. Since language is an ever-changing creature, we are sure that these terms will eventually be abbreviated in many languages but so far you can hear them referred to mostly as expanded terms:

NSCLC Non-small-cell lung cancer
PBSC   Peripheral blood stem cell

There is another group which we call the *energy-saving* abbreviations. These are abbreviations that many languages leave in the English original and, of course, when expanding them the first letter of each word doesn't match the abbreviation. We call them energy-saving because it wouldn't have been so difficult to come up with a real "national" abbreviation for that term. When looking for examples, we realized that most hormone names are energy-saving abbreviations:

FSH   Follicle-stimulating hormone
TNF   Tumor necrosis factor
PAW   Pulmonary arterial wedge

There is yet another kind, which we call the *double-meaning* abbreviations. This is when one abbreviation can refer to two different terms. The context helps, of course, to discern the real meaning. However, it is worth keeping an eye open for these because, if misinterpreted, these abbreviations might get you into an embarrassing situation:

- PCR
  - Polymerase chain reaction
  - Plasma clearance rate
  - Pathological complete response
  - Protein catabolic rate
- HEV
  - Human enteric virus
  - Hepatitis E virus
- PID
  - Pelvic inflammatory disease
  - Prolapsed intervertebral disc
- CSF
  - Colony-stimulating factor
  - Cerebrospinal fluid

The funniest abbreviations are those that become acronyms in which the pronunciation resembles a word that has nothing to do with the abbreviation's meaning. We call this group the *mind-blowing* abbreviations.

A *cabbage* in English is that nice vegetable known for its gasogenic properties. However, when an English-speaking surgeon says "This patient is a clear candidate for *cabbage*", he/she isn't talking about what the patient should have for lunch, but rather the type of surgery he/she is suggesting should be performed. Thus, *cabbage* is the colloquial way of referring to *CABG* (coronary artery bypass grafting).

If you happen to be eavesdropping in a corridor and you hear an oncologist saying "I think your patient needs a *chop*", you walk on down the corridor, wondering whether this new alternative therapy will consist of a pork or a lamb chop. But then you quickly realize that the specialist you were eavesdropping on was actually referring to a *CHOP* (a regimen of cyclophosphamide, hydroxydaunomycin, oncovin and prednisone, used in cancer chemotherapy).

There are more abbreviations out there, and there are also more to come. The medical profession is sure to keep us busy catching up with its incursions into linguistic creation.

Regardless of the "type" of abbreviation you have before you, we will give you three pieces of advice:

1. Identify the most common abbreviations.
2. Read the abbreviations in your lists.
3. Begin with abbreviation lists of your radiological subspecialty.

Read the abbreviations in your lists. Read the abbreviations in your lists in a natural way. Bear in mind that to be able to identify written abbreviations may not be enough. From this standpoint, there are three types of abbreviations:

1. Spelt abbreviations
2. Read abbreviations (acronyms)
3. Half-spelled/half-read abbreviations

Nobody would understand a spelt abbreviation if you read it and nobody would understand a read abbreviation if you spelt it. Let us make clear what we are trying to say with an example. LAM stands for lymphangiomyomatosis and must be read *lam*. Nobody would understand you if instead of saying *lam* you spell L-A-M. Therefore, never spell a "read abbreviation" and never read a "spelt abbreviation".

Most abbreviations are spelt abbreviations, and are usually those in which the letter order makes them almost impossible to read. Think, for example, of COPD (chronic obstructive pulmonary disease) and try to read the abbreviation instead of spelling it. Never use the "expanded form" (chronic obstructive pulmonary disease) of a classic abbreviation such as this one because it would sound extraordinarily unnatural.

Some abbreviations have become acronyms and therefore must be read and not spelt. Their letter order allows us to read them. LAM belongs to this group.

The third type is made up of abbreviations such as CPAP (continuous positive airway pressure) which is pronounced something like *C-pap*. If you spell out CPAP (C-P-A-P), nobody will understand you.

Review abbreviation lists on your specialty. Review as many abbreviation lists on your specialty as you can and double-check them until you are familiar with their meaning and pronunciation.

Although you should make your own abbreviation lists, we have created several classified by specialty. To begin with, check whether your own specialty's list is included; if not, start writing your own. Be patient ... this task can last the rest of your professional life.

Abbreviation Lists

General List

5FU	5-Fluorouracil
ABPA	Allergic bronchopulmonary aspergillosis
ACE	Angiotensin-converting enzyme
aCL	Antibodies to cardiolipin
ACTH	Adrenocorticotropic hormone
ADH	Antidiuretic hormone
ADPKD	Autosomal dominant polycystic kidney disease
AF	Atrial fibrillation
AFP	Alpha fetoprotein
AJCC	American Joint Cancer Commission
ALT	Alanine aminotransferase
α1AT	α1-Antitrypsin
AML	Acute myeloid leukemia
ANA	Antinuclear antibodies
APCs	Atrial premature complexes
API	Arterial pressure index
APUD	Amine precursor uptake and decarboxylation system
ARDS	Acute respiratory distress syndrome
ARF	Acute renal failure
AS	Ankylosing spondylitis
AST	Aspartate aminotransferase
ATN	Acute tubular necrosis
AVP	Arginine vasopressin
BAL	Bronchoalveolar lavage
BCC	Basal cell carcinoma

BCG	Bacillus Calmette-Guérin
BMT	Bone marrow transplant
BP	Bullous pemphigoid
BPF	Brazilian purpuric fever
CBD	Common bile duct
CCK	Cholecystokinin
CD	Crohn disease
CEA	Carcinoembryonic antigen
CF	Cystic fibrosis
CML	Chronic myeloid leukemia
CMML	Chronic myelomonocytic leukemia
COPD	Chronic obstructive pulmonary disease
CP	Cicatricial pemphigoid
CRF	Chronic renal failure
CRH	Corticotropin-releasing hormone
CSF	Colony stimulating factor
CT	Computed tomography
CTX	Cholera toxin
CUPS	Cancer of unknown primary site
CWP	Coal workers' pneumoconiosis
CXR	Chest X-ray
DCIS	Ductal carcinoma in situ
DLE	Discoid lupus erythematosus
DGI	Disseminated gonococcal infection
DH	Dermatitis herpetiformis
DISH	Diffuse idiopathic skeletal hyperostosis
DPB	Diastolic blood pressure
DRA	Dialysis-related amyloidosis
DRE	Digital rectal examination
DU	Duodenal ulcer
DVT	Deep venous thrombosis
EBA	Epidermolysis bullosa acquisita
EBV	Epstein Barr virus
ECG	Electrocardiogram
EGD	Esophagogastroduodenoscopy
ERCP	Endoscopic retrograde cholangiopancreatography
ESRD	End-stage renal disease
FAP	Familial amyloid polyneuropathies
FEV_1	Forced expiratory volume in one second
FMF	Familial Mediterranean fever
FSGS	Focal and segmental glomerulosclerosis
FSH	Follicle-stimulating hormone
GBM	Glomerular basement membrane
GCT	Germ cell tumor
GFR	Glomerular filtration rate
GGT	γ-Glutamyltranspeptidase, γ-glutamyltransferase

GH	Growth hormone
GHRH	Growth hormone-releasing hormone
GI	Gastrointestinal
GIP	Gastrin inhibitory peptide
GU	Gastric ulcer
HBV	Hepatitis B virus
hCG	Human chorionic gonadotropin
HCV	Hepatitis C virus
HIVAN	Human immunodeficiency virus-associated nephropathy
HOA	Hypertrophic osteoarthropathy
HP	Hypersensitivity pneumonitis
HPV	Human papilloma virus
HRT	Hormone replacement therapy
HSC	Hematopoietic stem cell
HUS	Hemolytic uremic syndrome
IBD	Inflammatory bowel disease
IBS	Irritable bowel syndrome
IL	Interleukin
ILD	Interstitial lung disease
IPSID	Immunoproliferative small intestinal disease (Mediterranean lymphoma)
ITP	Idiopathic thrombocytopenic purpura
JN	Juvenile nephronophthisis
LA	Lupus anticoagulant
LBBB	Left bundle branch block
LCDD	Light chain deposition disease
LDH	Lactate dehydrogenase
LES	Lower esophageal sphincter
LH	Luteinizing hormone
LIP	Lymphoid interstitial pneumonitis
MAC	*Mycobacterium avium* complex
MALT	Mucosa-associated lymphoid tissue
MCD	Medullary cystic disease
MCD	Minimal change disease
MCHC	Mean corpuscular hemoglobin concentration
MCTD	Mixed connective tissue disease
MCV	Mean corpuscular volume
MEN1	Type 1 multiple endocrine neoplasia
MPGN	Membranoproliferative glomerulopathies
MR	Magnetic resonance
MRI	Magnetic resonance imaging
NSAIDs	Nonsteroidal anti-inflammatory drugs
NUD	Non-ulcer dyspepsia
OA	Osteoarthritis
OCG	Oral cholecystography

ODTS	Organic dust toxic syndrome
OSA	Obstructive sleep apnea
PAH	Primary alveolar hypoventilation
PAN	Polyarteritis nodosa
PAP	Pulmonary alveolar proteinosis
PBC	Primary biliary cirrhosis
PCI	Prophylactic cranial irradiation
PCP	*Pneumocystis carinii* pneumonia
PDR	Physicians' desk reference (vademecum)
PEG	Percutaneous endoscopic gastrostomy
PF	Pemphigus foliaceus
PG	Pemphigoid gestationis
PIF	Prolactin inhibitory factor
PML	Progressive multifocal leukoencephalopathy
PNET	Peripheral primitive neuroectodermal tumor
PRA	Plasma renin activity
PRL	Prolactin
PSA	Prostate-specific antigen
PsA	Psoriatic arthritis
PTC	Percutaneous transhepatic cholangiography
PTE	Pulmonary thromboembolism
PTH	Parathyroid hormone
PV	Pemphigus vulgaris
RA	Rheumatoid arthritis
RBBB	Right bundle branch block
RBC	Red blood cell
RF	Rheumatoid factor
RMSF	Rocky mountain spotted fever
RPGN	Rapidly progressive glomerulonephritis
RPRF	Rapidly progressive renal failure
RTA	Renal tubular acidosis
RV	Residual volume
RVT	Renal vein thrombosis
SBC	Secondary biliary cirrhosis
SBP	Systolic blood pressure
SCC	Squamous cell carcinoma
SCID	Severe combined immunodeficiency
SCLE	Subacute cutaneous lupus erythematosus
SI	Serum iron
SIADH	Syndrome of inappropriate secretion of antidiuretic hormone
SLE	Systemic lupus erythematosus
SPB	Spontaneous bacterial peritonitis
SSc	Systemic sclerosis
SVCS	Superior vena cava syndrome
TB	Tuberculosis

TBB	Transbronchial biopsy
TGFβ	Transforming growth factor β
TIBC	Transferrin iron-binding capacity
TIPS	Transjugular intrahepatic portosystemic shunt
TLC	Total lung capacity
TNF	Tumor necrosis factor
TRH	Thyrotropin-releasing hormone
TSH	Thyroid-stimulating hormone
TTA	Transtracheal aspiration
TTP	Thrombotic thrombocytopenic purpura
UC	Ulcerative colitis
US	Ultrasonography
VATS	Video-assisted thoracic surgery
VC	Vital capacity
VF	Ventricular fibrillation
VIP	Vasoactive intestinal peptide
VPCs	Ventricular premature complexes
WBC	White blood cell
WDHA syndrome	Watery diarrhea, hypokalemia and achlorhydria syndrome (Verner-Morrison)
ZES	Zollinger-Ellison syndrome

Lists by Specialty

Anatomy

AC	Acromioclavicular joint
ACL	Anterior cruciate ligament
ACS	Anterior cervical space
ARA	Anorectal angle
ATA	Anterior tibial artery
BNA	Basle Nomina Anatomica
CBD	Common bile duct
CFA	Common femoral artery
CHA	Common hepatic artery
CHD	Common hepatic duct
CN	Cranial nerve
CNS	Central nervous system
CS	Carotid space
DCF	Deep cervical fascia
DLDCF	Deep layer of the deep cervical fascia
DRUJ	Distal radioulnar joint
ECU	Extensor carpi ulnaris
EEL	External elastic lamina
GB	Gallbladder

GDA	Gastroduodenal artery
GE	Gastroesophageal junction
GI	Gastrointestinal
IANC	International anatomical nomenclature
ICA	Internal carotid artery
ICRP	International Commision on Radiological Protection
IEL	Internal elastic lamina
IHBD	Intrahepatic biliary ducts
IMA	Inferior mesenteric artery
ITB	Iliotibial band
IVC	Inferior vena cava
JV	Jugular vein
LA	Left atrium
LAA	Left atrial appendage
LAD	Left anterior descending coronary artery
LCL	Lateral collateral ligament
LCX	Left circumflex coronary artery
LES	Lower esophageal sphincter
LGA	Left gastric artery
LHA	Left hepatic artery
LHD	Left hepatic duct
LHV	Left hepatic vein
LIMA	Left internal mammary artery
LLL	Left lower lobe (of lung)
LLQ	Left lower quadrant (of abdomen)
LPV	Left portal vein
LUCL	Lateral ulnar collateral ligament
LUL	Left upper lobe (of lung)
LUQ	Left upper quadrant (of abdomen)
LV	Left ventricle
LVOT	Left ventricular outflow tract
MCL	Medial collateral ligament
MCP	Metacarpophalangeal
MHV	Middle hepatic artery
MLDCF	Middle layer of the deep cervical fascia
MS	Masticator space
MTP	Metatarsophalangeal
NA	Nomina anatomica
OM	Obtuse marginal branch
PCL	Posterior cruciate ligament
PCS	Posterior cervical space
PDA	Posterior descending anterior coronary artery, patent ductus arteriosus
PDV	Pancreaticoduodenal vein
PHA	Proper hepatic artery
PICA	Posteroinferior cerebellar artery

PMS	Pharyngeal mucosal space
PS	Parotid space
PTA	Posterior tibial artery
PV	Portal vein
RA	Right atrium
RAS	Reticular activating system
RCL	Radial collateral ligament
RDPA	Right descending pulmonary artery
RHA	Right hepatic artery
RHD	Right hepatic duct
RHV	Right hepatic vein
RIMA	Right internal mammary artery
RL	Right lower lobe (of lung)
RLQ	Right lower quadrant (of abdomen)
RPS	Retropharyngeal space
RPV	Right portal vein
RUL	Right upper lobe (of lung)
RUQ	Right upper quadrant (of abdomen)
RV	Right ventricle
RVOT	Right ventricular outflow tract
SCF	Superficial cervical fascia
SCM	Sternocleidomastoid muscle
SCV	Subclavian vein
SFA	Superficial femoral artery
SLS	Sublingual space
SMA	Superior mesenteric artery
SMC	Smooth muscle cell
SMS	Submandibular space
SMV	Superior mesenteric vein
ST	Scapulothoracic
STT	Scaphoid–trapezium–trapezoid
SVC	Superior vena cava
TE	Tracheoesophageal
TFCC	Triangular fibrocartilage complex
TMJ	Temporomandibular joint
TMT	Tarsometatarsal
UCL	Ulnar collateral ligament
UES	Upper esophageal sphincter
UPJ	Ureteropelvic junction
UVJ	Ureterovesical junction
VS	Visceral space

Clinical History

ABCD	Airway, breathing, circulation, defibrillate in cardio-pulmonary resuscitation
ABSYS	Above symptoms
AC, a.c.	Ante cibum (before a meal)
ad lib.	Ad libitum (as desired)
ADR	Adverse drug reaction
AU	Auris uterque (each ear)
AVPU	Alert, responsive to verbal stimuli, responsive to painful stimuli, and unresponsive (assessment of mental status)
AWS	Alcohol withdrawal symptoms
BC, BLCO, cbc	(Complete) blood count
BID, b.i.d.	Bis in die (twice a day)
BIO	Biochemistry
BIPRO	Biochemistry profile
BP	Blood pressure
BUCR	BUN and creatinine
BUN/Cr, BUCR	Blood urea nitrogen/creatinine
CC	Chief complaint
CCCR	Calculated creatinine clearance
Ch. D.	Chirugiae doctor, surgery doctor
Cib.	Cibus (food)
COEPS	Cortically originating extrapyramidal symptoms
CPE, CPX	Complete physical examination
CR	Creatinine
CrCl	Creatinine clearance
CVS	Current vital signs
d.	Dexter (right)
DD, D/D, DDX	Differential diagnosis
DIFFRLS	Differentials
DM	Diastolic murmur
DNR	Do not resuscitate
DOA	Dead on arrival
DRE	Digital rectal examination
DTR	Deep tendon reflex
E/A	Emergency admission
EAU	Emergency admission unit
EPMS	Extrapyramidal motor symptoms
ESR	Erythrocyte sedimentation rate
FCUS	First-catch urine sediment
FEN	Fluid, electrolytes, and nutrition
FH, FAHX	Family history
FH+/FH–	Family history positive/negative
FHA/FHHD	Family history of alcoholism/heavy drinking

FHCa	Family history of cancer
FHEH	Family history of essential hypertension
FHMI	Family history of mental illness
FHSF	Family history symptom free
FHVD	Family history of vascular disease
GERS	Gastroesophageal reflux symptoms
GISYS	Gastrointestinal symptoms
GP	General practitioner
H&P	History and physical examination
HARPPS	Heat, absence of use, redness, pain, pus, swelling
IBSY	Irritable bowel symptoms
IRSS	Illness-related symptoms
IV, i.v.	Intravenous
LUQ	Left upper quadrant (of abdomen)
LUTS	Lower urinary tract symptoms
M.D.	Medicinae doctor
MOUS	Mutiple occurrence of unexplained symptoms
NBM	Nil by mouth (nothing by mouth, U.K.)
NFH	Negative family history
NIS	No inflammatory signs
NNS	Non-specific symptoms
NOHF	No heart failure symptoms
NOSYS	No symptoms
NPO	Nil per os (nothing by mouth, U.S.)
NPx	Neurologist's physical examination
NSAD	No signs of acute disease
NSI	No signs of infection/inflammation
NVS	Neurological vital signs
NVS	No visual symptoms
OD	Oculus dexter (right eye), overdose
OPEX	On physical examination
OS	Oculus sinister (left eye)
p.c.	Post cibum (after meals)
p.r.n.	Pro re nata (according to circumstances, may require)
p.v.	Per vaginam
PC	Present complaint
PCA	Patient-controlled analgesia
PCLS	Persistent cold-like symptoms
PE, Pex, Px, PHEX	Physical examination
PESS	Problem, etiology, signs and symptoms
PFH	Positive family history
PH, PHx	Past history
PHI	Past history of illness
PMS	Premenstrual symptoms
PO, P.O.	Per os (by mouth, orally)
POMR	Problem-oriented medical record

PPES	Peer physical examinations
ppm	Parts per million
PRE	Progressive-resistance exercise
PS	Prescription
PT	Physical therapy/therapist
q.2h.	Quaque secunda hora (every two hours)
q.3h.	Quaque tertia hora (every three hours)
q.d.	Quaque die (every day)
q.h.	Quaque hora (every hour)
q.i.d.	Quater in die (four times daily)
q.v.	Quantum vis (as much as desired)
RBC	Red blood count
RDA	Recommended daily allowance
RESP	Respiratory symptoms
RLL	Right lower lobe (of lung)
RLQ	Right lower quadrant (of abdomen)
RML	Right middle lobe (of lung)
RMSD	Rheumatic-musculoskeletal symptoms/diseases
RS	Review of symptoms
RUL	Right upper lobe (of lung)
RUQ	Right upper quadrant (of abdomen)
Rx	Prescribe, prescription drug
S&S, S/S, SS	Signs and symptoms
SASR	Symptoms of acute stress reaction
SC, S/C, SQ	Subcutaneous
si op. sit,	si opus sit (if necessary)
SM	Systolic murmur
SOAP	Subjective, objective, assessment, and plan (used in problem-oriented records)
SSHF	Signs and symptoms of heart failure
SUS	Stained urinary sediment
Sx	Signs
t.i.d.	Ter in die (three times daily)
TFT	Thyroid function test
TINFHO/NFHO	(There is) no family history of ...
TPN	Total parenteral nutrition
TRINS	Totally reversible ischemic neurological symptoms
TWBC	(Total) white blood count
U&E	Urea and electrolytes
UEE	Urinary excretion of electrolytes
UGIS	Upper gastrointestinal symptoms
UGS	Urogenital symptoms
URELS	Urine electrolytes
VR	Vocal resonance
VS, vs	Vital signs
VSA	Vital signs absent

| VSOK | Vital signs normal |
| WRS | Work-related symptoms |

The Hospital

CCU	Coronary care unit
CCU	Critical care unit
ICF	Intermediate care facility
ICU	Intensive care unit
ECU	Emergency care unit
EMS	Emergency medical service
ER	Emergency room
OT	Operating theater/theatre

Radiology

Computed Tomography (CT), Image Reconstruction and Reformation

CAT	Computed axial tomography
CECT	Contrast enhanced CT
CPR	Curved planar reformation
CT	Computed tomography
CTA	CT angiography, CT arteriography
CTAP	CT during arterial portography
CTC	CT cholangiography
CTDI	CT dose index
CTHA	CT hepatic arteriography
CTM	CT myelography
CTP	CT perfusion imaging
CVS	Continuous volume scanning
DCTM	Delay CT myelography
DEQCT	Dual-energy quantitative CT
EBCT	Electron beam CT
EBT	Electron beam tomography
FOV	Field of view
FWAHM	Full width at half maximum
FWATA	Full width at tenth area
HRCT	High-resolution CT
HU	Hounsfield units
LI	Linear interpolation
MCTM	Metrizamide CT myelography
MIP	Maximum intensity projection
mIP, minIP	Minimum intensity projection
MLI	Multislice linear interpolation
MPR	Multiplanar reformation
MTT	Mean transit time

Nr-MIP	Noise-reduced maximum intensity projection
QCT	Quantitative CT
ROI	Region of interest
SC	Slice collimation
SEQCT	Single-energy CT
SFOV	Scan field of view
SNR	Signal-to-noise ratio
SSD	Shaded surface display
SSP	Section sensitiviy profile
SVS	Step volume scanning (EBCT)
TF	Table feed
UFCT	Ultrafast CT
VOI	Volume of interest
VRT	Volume rendering technique

Conventional Radiology

ABER	Abduction and external rotation
ACR	American College of Radiology
ALARA	As low as reasonably achievable (radiation dosages)
AP	Anteroposterior
ASNR	American Society of Neuroradiology
ASSR	American Society of Spine Radiology
At Wt, AW	Atomic Weight
BE	Barium enema
Bol	Bolus
Bq	Becquerel
BS	Barium swallow
C/C	Cholecystectomy and operative cholangiogram
CAG, CHGM	Cholangiogram
CAG, CHGRY	Cholangiography
CDG	Conventional dacryocystography
CPR	Curved planar reformation
CRT	Cathode ray tube
CSG, CG, CCG	Cholecystography or cholecystogram
CXR	Chest X-ray
DC	Double contrast
DCG	Dacryocystography
DCSA	Double-contrast shoulder arthrography
DFCG	Digital fluorocholangiogram
DICOM	Digital imaging and communications in medicine
DLP	Dose–length product
DSAR	Digital subtraction arthrography
FOV	Field of view
FWAHM	Full width at half maximum
FWATA	Full width at tenth area
H/S	Hysterosalpingography

HOCA	High osmolar contrast agent
ICRP	International Commision on Radiological Protection
IOCG	Intraoperative cholangiogram
IVCH	Intravenous cholangiogram
IVP	Intravenous pyelogram
IVU	Intravenous urogram
keV	Kiloelectron-volt
KUB	Kidney–ureters–bladder (plain abdominal radiography)
kV	Kilovolt
LAO	Left anterior oblique position
LAP	Late arterial phase
LMM	Lumbar metrizamide myelography
LOCM	Low osmolar contrast medium
LPO	Left posterior oblique position
LUT	Look-up table
MCU	Micturating cystography
MCUG	Micturating cystourethrogram
MLG	Myelography
Nr-MIP	Noise-reduced maximum intensity projection
OCC	Oral cholecystography
OCG	Oral cholangiogram
PA	Posteroanterior
PACS	Picture archive and communication system
PFMM	Plain film metrizamide myelography
PMG	Pneumomyelography
PS	Parotid sialography
PVP	Portal venous phase
RAO	Right anterior oblique
RC	Retrograde cystogram
RGPG, RGP	Retrograde pyelogram, retrograde pyelography
RGU, RUG	Retrograde urethrogram, retrograde urethrography
ROI	Region of interest
RPO	Right posterior oblique
RU	Retrograde urogram
RUP	Retrograde ureteropyelography, retrograde pyelogram
S/N, SNR	Signal to noise ratio
SBFT	Small-bowel follow-through examination
SC	Single contrast
SCGC	Single-contrast graded-compression technique (GI radiology)
SCVIR	Society of Cardiovascular and Interventional Radiology
SFOV	Scan field of view
SOL	Space-occupying lesion
SSD	Shaded surface display

TTC	T-tube cholangiogram
TTP	Time to peak
UCG, UCR	Urethrocystography
UGI	Upper gastrointestinal series
VCG	Voiding cystography
VCU, VCUG	Voiding cystourethrogram, voiding cystourethro- graphy
VOI	Volume of interest
VR	Volume rendering
VRT	Volume rendering technique
WSM	Water-soluble myelography
XR	X-ray

Interventional Radiology

BN	Bird's nest filter
CVA	Central venous access
DSA	Digital subtraction angiography
EAP	Early arterial phase
ERC	Endoscopic retrograde cholangiography
F	French (unit of a scale for denoting size of catheters)
FNAC	Fine-needle aspiration cytology
FWHM	Full width at half maximum
HDAF	Hemodynamic access fistula
IACB	Intraaortic counterpulsation balloon pump
LAP	Late arterial phase
LP	Lumbar puncture
PC	Percutaneous cholecystostomy
PCD	Percutaneous drainage
PCN	Percutaneous nephrostomy
PCWP	Pulmonary capillary wedge pressure
PEG	Percutaneous endoscopic gastrostomy
PEI	Percutaneous ethanol injection
PFG	Percutaneous fluoroscopic gastrostomy
PICC	Peripherally inserted central catheter
PTA	Percutaneous transluminal angioplasty
PTBD	Percutaneous transhepatic biliary drainage
PTC	Percutaneous transhepatic cholangiography
PTFE	Polytetrafluoroethylene
PTHC	Percutaneous transhepatic cholangiography
PVP	Portal venous phase, percutaneous vertebroplasty
Rt-PA	Recombinant tissue plasminogen activator
SCVIR	Standards of Practice Guidelines on Angioplasty
SK	Streptokinase
TACE	Transcatheter arterial chemoembolization
TIPS	Transjugular intrahepatic portosystemic shunt
TNB	Transthoracic needle biopsy

tPA	Tissue plasminogen activator
TTP	Time to peak
UK	Urokinase
VT	Vena-Tech (vena cava filter)

Magnetic Resonance Imaging (MRI)

CHESS	Chemical shift selective pulses
CME-MRI	Contrast medium-enhanced MRI
CNR	Contrast to noise ratio
COPE	Centrally ordered phase encoding
CSI	Chemical shift imaging (magnetic resonance spectroscopy method)
CVMR	Cardiovascular magnetic resonance
DNMR	Dynamic nuclear magnetic resonance
DTPA	Diethylene triamine pentaacetic acid (a binding substance for both Gd and 99m-Tc)
DWI	Diffusion-weighted image
EMRI	Electron MRI
EPI	Echoplanar imaging
EPMR	Echoplanar magnetic resonance
EP-MRSI	Echoplanar magnetic resonance spectroscopic imaging
ERSC-MRI	Endorectal surface coil MRI
ESR	Electron spin resonance
ETL	Echo train length
FAST	Fourier-acquired steady-state technique
FC	Flow compensation
FID	Free induction decay
FISP	Fast imaging with steady-state precession
FLASH	Fast low-angle shot
fMRI	Functional MRI
FMRIB	Functional MRI of the brain
FS	Fast saturation
FSE	Fast spin echo
FT	Fourier transform
FTNMR	Fourier transform nuclear magnetic resonance
Gd-DTPA	Gadolinium-diethylenetriamine penta-acetic acid
Gd-MRA	Gadolinium-enhanced magnetic resonance arteriography
GE	Gradient echo
GEMRA	Gadolinium-enhanced magnetic resonance angiography
GRASS	Gradient-recalled acquisition in steady-state
GRE	Gradient-recalled echo, gradient echo
GRM	Gradient rephasing motion
HASTE	Half Fourier acquisition single-shot turbo spin echo

i-MR	Interventional MRI
IR	Inversion recovery
ISMRM	International Society for Magnetic Resonance in Medicne
MAS NMR	Magic angle spinning nuclear magnetic resonance
MOTSA	Multiple overlapping thin-slab acquisition
MPGR	Multiplanar two-dimensional gradient echo
MRA	Magnetic resonance angiography
MRA	Magnetic resonance arthrography
MRCP	Magnetic resonance cholangiopancreatography
MRE	Magnetic resonance elastography, magnetic resonance enteroclysis
MRI	Magnetic resonance imaging
MRM	Magnetic resonance myelography
MRS	Magnetic resonance spectroscopy
MRU	Magnetic resonance urography
MRV	Magnetic resonance venography/venogram
MTF	Modulation transfer function
MTP	Magnetization transfer pulse
NAA	N-Acetyl aspartate (MR spectroscopy)
NAQ	Number of acquisitions
NEX	Number of excitations
NMRI	Nuclear MRI
PC	Phase contrast
PMR	Proton magnetic resonance
PWI	Perfusion-weighted imaging
RF	Radiofrequency
ROPE	Respiratory-ordered phase encoding
SAR	Specific absorption rate
SE	Spin echo
SENSE	Sensitivity encoding for MRI
SLS	Interslice spacing
SLTHK	Slice thickness
SMASH	Simultaneous acquisition of spatial harmonics
SMRI	Society of Magnetic Resonance Imaging
SPGR	Spoiled gradient recalled acquisition in steady state, spoiled gradient-recalled echo
SPIO	Superparamagnetic iron oxide (particles)
SPIR	Spectral presaturation by inversion recovery
SSFP	Steady-state free precession
SSNMR	Solid-state nuclear magnetic resonance
STEAM	Stimulated-echo acquisition mode
STIR	Short-tau inversion recovery, short T1 inversion recovery

T1w	T1-weighted image
T2w	T2-weighted image
TE	Time to echo (echo time)
TI	Inversion time
TOF	Time of flight
TR	Time of repetition (repetition time)
TSE	Turbo spin echo
USPIO	Ultrasmall superparamagnetic particles
VENC-MR	Velocity-encoded cine MRI

Nuclear Medicine

AXL	Axillary lymphoscintigraphy
CPDS	Computer processed dynamic scintigraphy
CS	Cerebral scintigraphy
DIC	Direct isotope cystography
DMSA	99m-Tc-Dimercaptosuccinic acid scintigraphy
DPLS	Dynamic perfusory lung scintigraphy
DRC, DRCG, DRNC	Direct radionuclide cystography
DRVC	Direct radionuclide voiding cystography
DTMS	Dipyridamole-Thallium myocardial scintigraphy
EMPS	Exercise myocardial perfusion scintigraphy
HBFS	Hepatobiliary functional scintigraphy
HIDA	Hepatobiliary scintigraphy with dimethylimino-diacetic acid
IMP	I-123-Isopropyliodoamphetamine (radiolabeled agent for brain perfusion SPECT)
IRC	Indirect radionuclide cystography
IVCU	Isotope-voiding cystourethrogram
MPS	Myocardial perfusion scintigraphy
PET	Positron emission tomography
rCBF	Regional cerebral blood flow
RIA	Radioimmunoassay
RNVC, RNC	Radionuclide voiding cystography
SCINT	Scintigraphy
SESC	Sestamibi scan
SPECT	Single photon emission computed tomography
SRS	Somatostatin receptor scintigraphy
SSMM	Sestamibi scintimammography
Tc-99m-ECD-bicisate	Technetium-99m bicisate ethyl cysteinate dimer (radiolabeled agent for brain perfusion SPECT)
Tc-99m-HMPAO	Technetium-99m-hexamethyl propylamine oxime (radiolabeled agent for Brain Perfusion SPECT)
Tc-99mI-123-QNB	Technetium-99m-iodine-123-quinuclidinyl-iodo-benzylate
Tc-99m-labeled RBCs	Red blood cell scan (Meckel's scan)
TMS	Thalium myocardial scintigraphy

TPBS	Three-phase dynamic bone scintigraphy
V/Q scanning	Ventilation-perfusion scintigraphy
WBC scans	White blood cell scans
WBS	Whole body scintigraphy
WCS	White cell scintigraphy

Ultrasonography

3D-US	Three-dimensional ultrasound
AD	Acoustic densitometry (ultrasound)
B-mode	Brightness-mode
BPD	Bi-parietal diameter (ultrasound measurement of the head of a fetus)
CCUS	Complete compression ultrasound
CDI	Color Doppler imaging
CEUS	Contrast-enhanced ultrasound
CRL	Crown rump length (ultrasound fetal measurement)
CW Doppler	Continuous wave Doppler
DPVTI	Doppler power velocity time integral
DR	Dynamic range
EDV	End diastolic velocity
EFOV	Extended field of view
EJU	European Journal of Ultrasound
ELB	Echolucent band
ERUS, EUS	Endorectal ultrasonography, endorectal ultrasound
ESB	Echostrong band
EUS	Endovascular ultrasonography, endoscopic ultrasound
EVS	Endovaginal sonography
EVUS	Endovaginal ultrasound
ISUOG	International Society of Ultrasound in Obstetrics and Gynecology
IVUS	Intravascular ultrasound
PDI	Power Doppler imaging
PI	Pulsatility index
PIM	Pulse inversion mode
PNU	Prenatal ultrasonography
PRF	Pulse repetition frequency
PSV	Peak systolic velocity
PWD	Pulsed-wave Doppler
QUI	Quantitative ultrasound index (bone density)
QUS	Quantitative ultrasound
RI	Resistivity index
RTU	Real-time ultrasound
SVU	Society for Vascular Ultrasound
TAUS	Transabdominal ultrasonography
TEE	Transesophageal echocardiography
TGC	Time-gain compensation

THI	Time harmonic imaging
TRUS	Transrectal ultrasound
TULIP	Transurethral ultrasound-guided laser-induced prostatectomy
TUS	Transabdominal ultrasound
US, USG	Ultrasound, ultrasonography
USB	Ultrasound-guided aspiration biopsy
USMF	Ultrasound multi-frame (images)
VUS	Voiding urosonography, voiding urethrosonography

Exercises: Common Sentences Containing Abbreviations

This section presents common sentences containing abbreviations, followed by the definitions of the abbreviations used.

Sentences:

- A 40-year-old man visited our hospital, and was diagnosed as having Felty's syndrome because of splenomegaly and pancytopenia as well as definite RA.
- MCV, MCHC, LDH, ANA and RF values are normal.
- The platelet and WBC counts exceeded their normal ranges. He was diagnosed as suffering from ... (ITP, CMML, AML, CML). Two months after, he received a BMT.
- Foreign bodies display a variable signal intensity on both T1- and T2-weighted images. MR shows an inflammatory response while CT can show the retained foreign body. US evaluation could be useful in selected patients.
- COPD is a risk factor in the development of TB.
- Cholera can be diagnosed by the presence of CTX in stools.
- A 16-year-old female suffering from fever, chills, rash and presenting multiple nodular opacities in CXR was diagnosed as having ... (RMSF, BPF, DGI).
- An ECG was obtained, and showed ... (RBBB, LBBB, APCs, VPCs, AF, VF).
- He is actually under treatment with ACEI. Ten years ago he was treated with PTCA because of the three AMI he had suffered.
- RA and SSc are more common in females.
- PCP and PML are two of the complications that can be suffered by AIDS patients.

- Cutaneous manifestations of SLE can be divided into SCLE (acute) and DLE (chronic).
- The key to the diagnosis of septic arthritis is joint aspiration. Joint fluid is opaque and has a WBC count greater than 100,000.
- Clinical signs of skeletal metastases include hypercalcemia and the syndrome known as HPO.
- Prolonged morning stiffness helps to distinguish a truly inflammatory arthritis such as RA from non-inflammatory arthritides such as OA.
- The typical attack of acute gouty arthritis is a painful monoarthritis, most often in the first MTP joint (podagra).
- Scaphoid fractures exhibit a high rate of non-union and AVN.
- Water is arbitrarily assigned a value of 0 HU.
- MRI is the imaging modality of choice for the CNS.
- The aorta is normally visible on PA and lateral chest radiographs.
- Generally, a PT of below 15 seconds, a PTT within 1.2 times control and a platelet count greater than 75,000/ml will be acceptable.
- TIPS is a relatively new technique for the treatment of patients with portal hypertension.
- To rule out the presence of DVT, a lower extremity ultrasound examination should be performed.
- Approximately 1% of cardiac muscle cells, including those in the SA and AV nodes, are autorhythmic.
- In the chronic form of mitral regurgitation, clinical monitoring focuses on the evaluation of left ventricular function, with treatment of CHF.
- The RCA supplies the right ventricle and the AV node.
- The LCA divides into the anterior descending and circumflex arteries.
- In the ARDS an increase in capillary permeability occurs.
- SOB can usually be attributed to one of two fundamental categories of disease, cardiac or pulmonary.
- In patients with documented DVT or PE in whom anticoagulation is contraindicated, percutaneous placement of an IVC filter in the angiography suite may be warranted.
- The azygous vein provides venous drainage into the SVC.
- NHL carries a less-favorable prognosis than Hodgkin's disease.
- There is a strong association between thymoma and MG.
- Neurofibromas and schwannomas are more common in patients with NF-1.
- KS remains the most common malignancy in HIV disease and constitutes an AIDS-defining illness.
- LIP is an AIDS-defining illness in children.
- One of the classic differential diagnoses in radiology is that of the SPN.
- The SMA supplies the bowel between the duodenojejunal junction and the splenic flexure of the colon.
- CT scanning has replaced DPL for detecting and evaluating free fluid within the abdominal cavity.
- The pelvis joins the ureter at the UPJ, a common site of obstruction.

- The higher incidence of UTIs in young women is attributed to the relatively short female urethra.
- When an ACE inhibitor is administered, glomerular filtration is reduced.
- Intrinsic renal causes of acute renal failure include ATN and acute glomerulonephritis.
- A clue to the prerenal nature of the failure is contained in the ratio of serum BUN to creatinine.
- The standard screening mammogram includes two views of each breast: the CC view and the MLO view.
- Hydrocephalus is called obstructive when there is a blockage of normal flow of CSF.
- Fetal growth is assessed by measurement of abdominal circumference, which is important in detecting IUGR.
- The transitional zone represents the site of BPH.
- Strokes are sometimes preceded clinically by so-called TIAs.
- The most common location of stroke is in the MCA distribution.
- ACA occlusion may cause contralateral foot and leg weakness.
- A small infarction in some portions of the PCA territory may have catastrophic consequences.
- HMD is the most common cause of neonatal respiratory distress.
- An important complication of long-term ventilatory support is BPD.
- TTN occurs when there is inadequate or delayed clearance of the fluid at birth, resulting in a "wet lung".
- EA and TEF both represent anomalies in the development of the primitive foregut.
- NEC occurs primarily in premature neonates exposed to hypoxic stress.
- DDH is suspected clinically in newborns with a breech presentation.
- PVL is the result of prenatal or neonatal hypoxic-ischemic insult.
- An AVM is a congenital lesion resulting from persistent fetal capillaries.

Definitions:

ACA	Anterior cerebral artery
ACE	Angiotensin-converting enzyme
ACEI	Angiotensin-converting enzyme inhibitor
AF	Atrial fibrillation
AIDS	Acquired immunodeficiency syndrome
AMI	Acute myocardial infarction
AML	Acute myeloid leukemia
ANA	Antinuclear antibodies
APCs	Atrial premature complexes
ARDS	Acute respiratory distress syndrome
ATN	Acute tubular necrosis
AV	Atrioventricular
AVM	Arteriovenous malformation
AVN	Avascular necrosis

BMT	Bone marrow transplantation
BPD	Bronchopulmonary dysplasia
BPF	Brazilian purpuric fever
BPH	Bening prostatic hyperplasia
BUN	Blood-urea nitrogen
CC	Craniocaudal
CHF	Congestive heart failure
CML	Chronic myeloid leukemia
CMML	Chronic myelomonocytic leukemia
CNS	Central Nervous System
COPD	Chronic obstructive pulmonary disease
CSF	Cerebrospinal fluid
CT	Computed tomography
CTX	Cholera toxin
CXR	Chest X-ray
DDH	Developmental dysplasia of the hip
DGI	Disseminated gonococcal infection
DLE	Discoid lupus erythematosus
DPL	Diagnostic peritoneal lavage
DVT	Deep venous thrombosis
EA	Esophageal atresia
ECG	Electrocardiogram
HIV	Human immunodeficiency virus
HMD	Hyaline membrane disease
HPO	Hypertrophic pulmonary osteoarthropaty
HU	Hounsfield units
ITP	Idiopathic thrombocytopenic purpura
IUGR	Intrauterine growth retardation
IVC	Inferior vena cava
KS	Kaposi's sarcoma
LBBB	Left bundle branch block
LCA	Left coronary artery
LDH	Lactate dehydrogenase
LIP	Lymphocytic interstitial pneumonitis
MCA	Middle cerebral artery
MCHC	Mean corpuscular hemoglobin concentration
MCV	Mean corpuscular volume
MG	Myasthenia gravis
MLO	Mediolateral oblique
MR	Magnetic resonance
MRI	Magnetic resonance imaging
MTP	Metatarsophalangeal
NEC	Necrotizing enterocolitis
NF-1	Neurofibromatosis type 1
NHL	Non-Hodgkin's lymphoma
OA	Osteoarthritis

PA	Posteroanterior
PCA	Posterior cerebral artery
PCP	*Pneumocystis carinii* pneumonia
PE	Pulmonary embolism
PML	Progressive multifocal leukoencephalopathy
PT	Prothrombin time
PTCA	Percutaneous transluminal coronary angioplasty
PTT	Partial thromboplastin time
PVL	Periventricular leukomalacia
RA	Rheumatoid arthritis
RBBB	Right bundle branch block
RCA	Right coronary artery
RF	Rheumatoid factor
RMSF	Rocky mountain spotted fever
SA	Sinoatrial
SCLE	Subacute cutaneous lupus erythematosus
SLE	Systemic lupus erythematosus
SMA	Superior mesenteric artery
SOB	Shortness of breath
SPN	Solitary pulmonary nodule
SSc	Systemic sclerosis
SVC	Superior vena cava
TB	Tuberculosis
TEF	Tracheoesophageal fistula
TIA	Transient ischemic attack
TIPS	Transjugular intrahepatic portosystemic shunting
TTN	Transient tachypnea of the newborn
UPJ	Ureteropelvic junction
US	Ultrasonography
UTI	Urinary tract infection
VF	Ventricular fibrillation
VPCs	Ventricular premature complexes
WBC	White blood cell

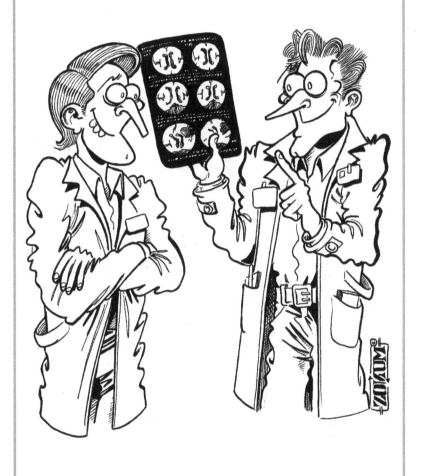

Unit XI   Describing a Lesion

Describing Anatomical Relationships

The description of the anatomical relationships of radiological findings is a problem for radiologists even in their own native tongues. To be able to talk properly on anatomical relationships you have, firstly, to have a sound knowledge of the anatomical structures and, secondly, to know certain anatomical expressions and phrasal verbs usually forgotten long time ago because many years have passed since we studied Anatomy at Medical School.

- Lesions can be *medial to* the medial collateral ligament, *cephalad to* the atriocaval junction, *caudal to* the cecum, *lateral to* the tail of the pancreas ...

To be cephalad/caudal/lateral to or *to be in relation with* are some of the indispensable phrasal verbs in Anatomy.

Let us think about this short anatomical paragraph:

- The scaphoid is the largest bone of the first carpal row. It is situated at the superior and external part of the carpus, its direction being from above downwards, outwards, and forwards. Its superior surface is convex, smooth, of triangular shape, and articulates with the lower end of the radius.

Anatomical literature is tremendously cumbersome. We, as radiologists, do not need to be so precise with regard to anatomical details, but we do need to be as precise as possible regarding the anatomical relationships of the radiological findings described in our reports.

Let us think now about this short radiological paragraph and notice how many anatomical words and collocations are used:

- Adenoma with ipsilateral stalk movement. There is a microadenoma present on the left side of the gland extending inferiorly and laterally. This case is unusual in that the stalk is displaced toward the side of the adenoma.

Anatomy and Radiology are intrinsically linked in radiological descriptions since we cannot describe a pituitary gland adenoma without talking about the pituitary gland itself, the stalk, the sella, the carotid arteries, the optic chiasm, the cavernous sinus ...

We can occasionally find difficulties with the spelling of some anatomical structures – was it gray mater or gray matter, was it dura mater or dura matter? (gray matter and dura mater) – or with the pronunciation of some terms – was "hippo" in hippocampus pronounced as "hypo" in hypothalamus? (No) – but, generally speaking, most radioanatomical difficulties are found in collocations and phrasal verbs such as "to give off":

- Previous to its division into the gastroepiploica dextra and the pancreaticoduodenalis, the gastroduodenalis artery *gives off* two or three small inferior pyloric branches to the pyloric end of the stomach and pancreas.

Let us analyze the following two-line sentence of anatomical English extracted without alteration from a musculoskeletal radiology article:

- The *elbow* is a *synovial hinge joint* between the *trochlea* and the *capitellum, articulating with* the *trochlear notch* of the *ulna* and the *radial head.*

More than half the words of the sentence come from Latin/Greek.

There are:
- One anatomical prepositional verb:
  – articulate *with*

- Three anatomical concepts containing more than one word:
  – synovial hinge joint
  – trochlear notch
  – radial head

- Two Anglo-Saxon anatomical nouns:
  – elbow
  – joint

- Three Latin/Greek nouns:
  – trochlea
  – capitellum
  – ulna

- Three Latin/Greek adjectives:
  – synovial
  – trochlear
  – radial

Imagine an English-speaking lay person in radiology trying to understand the sentence. The result would be something like:

- The elbow is a ... hinge joint between the ... and the ..., articulating with the ... notch of the ... and the ... head.

If you cannot also pronounce properly, what will be understood of your message will be something not too different from:

- The elbow is a ?? hinge joint between the ?? and the ??, articulating with the ?? notch of the ?? and the ?? head.

It is quite obvious that this sentence, without filling in the blanks, has no sense at all.

Although the need for a certain knowledge of Latin/Greek is, in principle, good news for health-care professionals from idiomatically Latin/Greek countries and bad news for those with native tongues that do not come from Latin/Greek, paradoxically many Latin doctors find great difficulty in pronouncing Latin/Greek terms in English, and for them Latin becomes an enemy instead of an ally. It is in the pronunciation of Latin terms where I can identify a colleague of my country as a Spaniard, although he/she speaks otherwise perfect English because it is very difficult to pronounce in English words as usual in our native tongue as edema or lipoma. I have noticed that sometimes Asian doctors, whose native tongues do not come from Latin/Greek, make fewer mistakes pronouncing Latin/Greek terms in English than their colleagues whose native languages have a great deal of Latin/Greek etymology.

- *Gross anatomy* specimen of the anterior aspect of the elbow joint.
    - *Gross anatomy* refers to macroscopic anatomy as opposed to the terms *microscopic* and *radiological anatomy*.

- The *lateral aspect* of the trochlea.
    - Although the lateral trochlea is colloquially acceptable and commonly used, the use of *lateral aspect* is more appropriate as there is only one trochlea in the elbow.

- The *medial aspect* of the olecranon
    - Similarly, the use of *medial aspect* is better than *medial* olecranon as there is only one olecranon in the elbow.

- The capsule is *attached* to the humeral head
    - The phrasal verb is "to be attached *to*". To be attached *at* is not acceptable.

- The triangular ulnar collateral ligament of the elbow *consists* of three strong bands.
    - To *consist of* is commonly used in anatomy to describe parts of a certain structure.

- The posterior band *extends from* the medial epicondyle *to* the *medial aspect* of the olecranon.
  - To *extend from ... to* is one of the most common phrasal verbs in anatomical English.

- The *medial epicondyle* is the last to fuse.
  - *Medial epicondyle* is a funny term since the prefix "epi" means above and the "medial epicondyle" is above the trochlea so, why don't name it "epitrochlea" as in some romance languages?

- *Pronation* and *supination* take place at the *proximal* and *distal* radioulnar joints.
  - To pronate and to supinate are typical anatomical verbs (pronation and supination are substantives) that describe upper limb movements.

- The annular ligament is the key structure of the proximal radioulnar joint *encircling* the radial head and neck without radial *attachment*.
  - *Encircling* an anatomical structure means to surround it without being *attached to* it.

- The conjoined insertion of the triceps muscle demonstrates low signal intensity at its attachment to the *posterosuperior* surface of the olecranon.
  - Posterosuperior, posteroinferior, posterolateral are preferred to superoposterior, inferoposterior, and lateroposterior.
  - Anterosuperior, anteroinferior, anterolateral are preferred to superoanterior, inferoanterior, and lateroanterior.

- The triceps muscle and tendon *are* located *posterior* **to.**
  - *To be posterior (anterior, lateral, caudal, cephalad, proximal,* and *distal) to* is one of the most common anatomical/radiological phrasal verbs. Posterior (anterior, lateral, caudal, cephalad, proximal, and distal) **at** is not acceptable.

Common Expressions in Vascular Anatomy

- The pulmonary artery *arises from* the right ventricle.
- The aorta *conveys* the oxygenated blood to every part of the body.
- The aorta *commences* at the upper part of the left ventricle.
- The arch of the aorta *extends from* the origin of the vessel to the lower border of the body of the third dorsal vertebra.
- The artery *describes a curve,* the convexity of which is directed upwards and to the right side.
- The ascending part of the aorta *is about two inches in length.*
- It *passes obliquely upwards* in the direction of the heart axis.
- The right coronary artery *sends a large branch* along the thin margin of the right ventricle to the apex.

- The left coronary artery *arises* immediately above the free edge of the left semilunar valve.
- The left coronary artery *divides into* two branches.
- The left coronary artery *supplies* the left auricle, both ventricles ...
- The innominate artery is the largest branch *given off from* the arch of the aorta.
- The left common carotid *lies on* the trachea, esophagus, and thoracic duct.
- The external carotid artery gives off eight branches which may be divided in four sets.
- The lingual artery *runs obliquely upwards and inwards* to the hyoid bone.

(Anatomical) Relations

- In front
- Behind
- On the right side
- On the left side
- Internally (medially)
- Externally (laterally)
- The ascending part of the arch is covered *at its commencement* by the trunk of the pulmonary artery and the right auricular appendage, and higher up, is separated from the sternum by the pericardium.
- *On the right side*, the ascending part of the aorta *is in relation with* the superior vena cava and right auricle.

Describing Radiological Findings: Word Order

Lesions have shape, borders, density, signal intensity, echogenicity, size, aggressive or non-aggressive aspect, and many other features.

How should we describe lesions, taking into account that we must use many adjectives?

Let us review these radiological descriptions:

- This sagittal image shows an ovoid hyperintense mass directly anterior to the infundibulum.
- A lateral radiograph shows a sclerotic, bubbly lesion in the anterior tibial shaft.
- T1-weighted axial images demonstrate a well-circumscribed low signal intensity tumor with intact overlying cortex.

In most radiological sentences we use fact adjectives (size, length), although sometimes we include opinion adjectives such as "aggressive" based on certain radiological features.

As a general rule opinion adjectives go before fact adjectives.
When several fact adjectives coexist in a sentence we put them in the following order:

1. Size/length
2. Shape/width
3. Age (generally not applicable; sometimes used in mentioning a previously described lesion)
4. Color (signal intensity, echogenicity, radiological density ...)
5. Material (bone, muscle, fat ...)

- A 5-cm (1), rounded (2), hyperintense on T2WI (4) fatty (5) lesion was found in the left lobe of the liver.

Describing Focal Lesions

It is far from our intention to offer a comprehensive set of checklists to be followed when reporting in English. Our only, and humble, goal is to provide you with a few useful idiomatic tools that can help you in your first reports in English.

From a radiological point of view these terms are easy and almost every radiologist has known them for many years. But to have them compiled in a couple of pages will save you time and allow you to concentrate on what is really important: the radiological findings themselves.

Since describing focal lesions in a radiological report can be troublesome for a non-native radiologist because of the scarcity of idiomatic resources, to count on an established description pattern is paramount.

These are some aspects you must not forget when describing a focal lesion. This is a standard checklist that can be used for any lesion, although some points are specific depending on the organ in which the lesion is sited:

1. **Solitary/single** or **multiple**: If multiple, the pattern of distribution may be reported (diffuse, segmental, lobar ...).
2. **Size** (large, small): Describe the size in millimeters. If multiple, you may mention the largest one and the smallest one.
3. **Shape** (round, oval, lobulated, irregular).
4. **Contour** (smooth, irregular) and **delimitation** from the adjacent parenchyma (well-delimited/defined, poorly/ill delimited/defined).
5. **Location**: Describing the location of focal lesions depends on the organ where they are sited.

- *Liver*: right hepatic lobe (segments V, VI, VII, VIII), left hepatic lobe (segments II, III, IVA, IVB), Caudate lobe (segment I). Another way of describing where focal lesions are sited is: anterior/posterior aspect of the RHL, LHL, and dome of the liver.
- *Pancreas*: the location can be divided into head, uncinate process, body and tail of the pancreas.
- *Kidney*: we refer to upper, mid or lower portions of the kidney. Upper pole or lower pole can also be used. The use of mid-pole is somewhat contradictory since poles mean extremes, but nonetheless "mid-pole" is extensively used.
- *Lung*: in the lung we locate the lesion according to the lobe (RUL, RLL, ML, LUL, LLL) and sometimes to the segment (the segments can be designated either anatomically or by numbers. There are two classical numerical classifications, the radiological and that of thoracic surgeons which basically differ in upper lobe segments 2 and 3). A few small details must be borne in mind when reporting lung lesions:
  - Don't forget that the expression right middle lobe is redundant since there is no left middle lobe since the lingula belongs to the left upper lobe.
  - Don't forget that segments IV and V belong to the middle lobe in the right lung and the lingula to the left lobe, but segment IV is beside segment V in the middle lobe and above segment V in the lingula.
  - Don't forget that segment VII (anterior, medial, and basal) does not exist as such in the left lung (some authors talk about segment VII–VIII).
- *CNS*: intracranial lesions can be either intraaxial or extraaxial. Intraaxial: cerebrum (frontal, temporal, parietal, and occipital lobes, and corpus callosum), brain stem, and cerebellum. Extraaxial: dura mater, arachnoid, or pia mater.
- *Spine* lesions can be divided into intradural intramedullary, intradural extramedullary and extradural.

6. **Density:**
  - Homogeneous/heterogeneous
  - Low/high density/intensity
  - Cystic/solid/complex (US)
  - Search for the presence of other different densities within the lesion: calcifications, fat, blood, necrosis, capsule, septa, scar.

7. **Enhancement** (enhancing lesion, non-enhancing lesion) and **pattern of enhancement:**
  - Evaluation in:
    - Arterial phase/portal venous phase/equilibrium phase/delayed phase (liver).
    - Arterial phase/corticomedullary phase/nephrographic phase/excretory phase (kidney). Plus, delayed phase if bladder needs to be evaluated.

    – Arterial phase/portal venous phase (rest of abdomen).

    – Arterial phase/venous phase (brain).

- Describing the enhancement:
  - Early enhancement vs. delayed enhancement
  - Diffuse homogeneous vs diffuse heterogeneous
  - Peripheral vs. central
  - Peripheral nodular vs. peripheral rim-like
  - Centripetal filling
  - Enhancing capsule/enhancing scar/enhancing septa
  - Enhancing satellite nodules
  - Early/delayed wash-out

8. Relations:

- Extension:
  - Superiorly, inferiorly, laterally, medially, anteriorly, posteriorly
- Displacement of adjacent structures:
  - Superiorly, inferiorly, medially, laterally, anteriorly, posteriorly
- Invasion, compression or encasement of adjacent structures
  - Arteries, veins, biliary tree and gallbladder, pelvocaliceal system, brain stem ...

9. Specific findings to look for:

- *Liver*: Search for: portal vein thrombosis, biliary tree dilation, gallbladder invasion, invasion of adjacent parenchyma, capsular retraction, hilar adenopathy, satellite lesions
- *Pancreas*: Search for: splenic vein thrombosis, Wirsung dilatation, distal common bile duct dilatation, peripancreatic/retroperitoneal adenopathy
- *Kidney*: Search for: renal vein thrombosis, pelvocaliceal distortion/dilation, ureteral dilatation, hilar and retroperitoneal adenopathy, perirenal fat involvement
- *Brain*: Search for: midline shift, ventricular dilatation/compression, brain stem displacement, cerebral herniation, hemorrhage, arterial encasement and secondary infarction, extraaxial lesions
- *Lung*: Search for: atelectasis, distal consolidation (pneumonitis), hilar and mediastinal adenopathy, hilar or mediastinal direct invasion, pleural effusion, chest wall invasion, pericardial invasion
- *Bone*: Search for: cortical destruction, cortical expansion, periosteal reaction, soft tissue mass, encasement/infiltration of neurovascular bundles

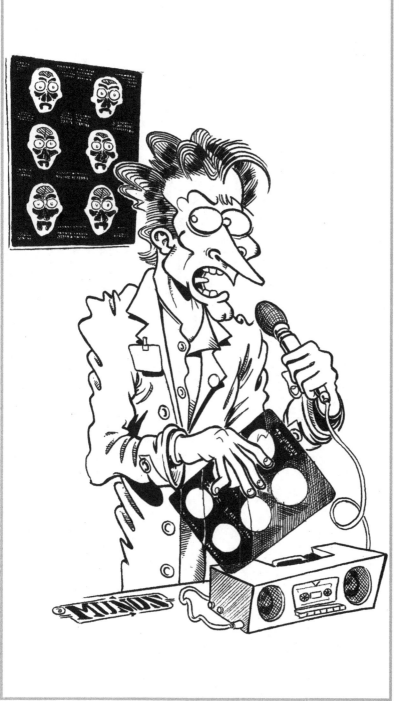

Unit XII Standard Normal Reports

In the old days, reporting in English was not an issue for most non-native English-speaking radiologists who, although they could read articles in English, would never report in a language other than their own. Things have changed so dramatically with the advent of tele-radiology that any well-trained radiologist in any country of the world would potentially be expected to report in English.

Medical reports communicate radiological findings and are legal documents. They should be logical, concise, and precise. Most reports end with the radiological impression in which a summary of the most relevant information is included. As a general rule, the most important information should be given first.

We have written two Units concerning radiological reports; this one reviews some of the most common normal radiological reports and Unit XIII is intended to provide some tips and idiomatic tools that may help when facing your first reports in English.

The first step in reporting in English is to start with normal reports. "Cruciate ligaments are unremarkable" must be one of the first sentences to be learnt if you want to report a knee MR scan because most cruciate ligaments are not injured (although many radiologists insist that the anterior cruciate ligament is partially torn, this being a historical discussion between radiologists and orthopedic surgeons who rarely see a partially torn anterior cruciate ligament and are unable, by means of arthroscopy, to see any intrasubstantial lesion).

In this unit we present some of the most common standard normal radiological reports and, in the last section called "Your First Radiological Reports in English", a "pluripathological" report in which both normal findings and the most common pathological findings are included.

Standard Reports

The standard radiological report is made up of the following sections:

1. History
2. Technique
3. Findings
4. Impression

In the following sections we present a selection of standard reports. Read them aloud and write them down and you will immediately notice which words deserve a greater amount of your attention regarding spelling and pronunciation (was it *intususception* or *intussusception*; *silhouete* or *silhouette*?).

CXR (Chest Radiograph)

- History:
  - Shortness of breath and fever.

- Findings:
  - Chest PA and lateral compared with similar study dated 6 September 2005 shows normal cardiomediastinal silhouette. The costophrenic sulci are sharp. The lungs are clear. There has been no significant interval change since the prior examination.

- Impression:
  - Normal chest radiograph.

KUB (Kidney Ureter and Bladder)

(KUB is the usual term for conventional abdominal radiographs.)

- History:
  - Abdominal pain.

- Findings:
  - Abdominal series consisting of supine and upright radiographs of the abdomen shows unremarkable bowel gas pattern. There is no evidence of free intraperitoneal air. No abnormal calcification or gas distribution is seen.

- Impression:
  - Unremarkable abdominal series with no findings to suggest an obstructive process or free intraperitoneal air.

UGI (Upper Gastrointestinal)

- History:
  - Abdominal pain.
- Technique:
  - Double contrast UGI study is performed by administration of thick and thin barium. Real-time fluoroscopic examination is complimented with spot images and overhead radiographs.
- Findings:
  - Patient is able to swallow without difficulty. Contrast material coating of the esophagus, stomach and duodenal bulb shows no ulceration or abnormal contour. The esophagus is of normal caliber. Contrast material transits into the stomach and duodenum unobstructed. Peristaltic waves are observed. The esophagus, stomach and duodenal bulb are pliable. No hiatal hernia is seen. Provocative maneuvers do not elicit gastroesophageal reflux.
- Impression:
  - Normal UGI study.

Barium Enema

- Clinical history:
  - Recent forty pound weight loss.
- Findings:
  - Normal ascending, transverse, descending, and sigmoid colon, and rectum with no evidence of stricture or mass. Contrast material refluxed into normal-appearing terminal ileum.
- Impression:
  - Normal.

Mammogram

- History:
  - Screening mammogram.
- Technique:
  - Standard mammographic views are obtained in the MLO and CC projection with digital mammography. CAD is applied. There is no prior mammogram for comparison. This is a baseline mammogram.

- Findings:
  - Bilateral breasts: there are scattered fibroglandular densities. No significant calcification, architectural distortion or mass is seen.

- Impression:
  - BIRADS 1 – normal.

Breast Sonography

- Clinical history:
  - Palpable mass and area of diffuse palpable nodularity.

- Findings:
  - Examination reveals no evidence of focal mass or cyst. Images compatible with focal fibroglandular tissue are noted.

- Impression:
  - No sonographic correlation with mammographic/palpable findings.

Chest CT Scan

- History:
  - Shortness of breath.

- Technique:
  - Multiple axial images of the chest from the thoracic inlet to the upper abdomen are acquired without intravenous contrast material. 5-mm contiguous axial images are reconstructed. There is no prior CT of the chest for comparison.

- Findings:
  - There is no axillary, mediastinal or hilar lymphadenopathy. The lungs are clear. Cardiac size within normal limits. No pericardial or pleural effusion is present. Imaged bones and soft tissues are unremarkable.

- Impression:
  - Normal chest CT scan.

Abdomen/Pelvis CT Scan

- History:
  - LUQ pain.

- Technique:
  - Multiple axial images of the abdomen and pelvis from the lung bases to the ischial tuberosities are acquired in coordination with intravenous administration of 100 ml [contrast agent] and oral contrast agent. 5-mm contiguous axial images are reconstructed. There is no prior CT of the abdomen/pelvis for comparison.

- Findings:
  - Lung bases are clear.
  - *Abdomen*: Liver has normal contour and density. Spleen, pancreas, adrenal glands and gallbladder are unremarkable. Kidneys enhance symmetrically. No lymph nodes in the abdomen are abnormally enlarged.
  - *Pelvis*: Opacified loops of large and small bowel are unremarkable. There is no free fluid in the pelvis. No lymph nodes are abnormally enlarged. The urinary bladder has a normal configuration.
  - No bony lesion is suspicious for malignancy.

- Impression:
  - Normal CT scan of the abdomen and pelvis.

Abdomen Ultrasonography

- History:
  - Right upper quadrant pain.

- Findings:
  - Real-time ultrasound examination of the abdomen shows normal liver contour and echotexture. The kidneys measure ...cm (left) and ...cm (right). Spleen and pancreatic head are unremarkable. The pancreatic tail is obscured by overlying bowel gas. The gallbladder is distended but no pericholecystic fluid or gallbladder wall thickening is present. No sonographic Murphy's sign could be elicited. The common bile duct measures 3 mm. There is no intra- or extrahepatic biliary ductal dilatation. The aorta diameter is 1.5 cm at the level of the renal arteries.

- Impression:
  - Normal abdominal ultrasound.

Head CT Scan

- History:
  - Headache.
- Technique:
  - Multiple axial images of the head are obtained from the skull base to the high convexities without administration of intravenous contrast agent. No similar prior study is available for comparison.
- Findings:
  - There is no intra- or extraaxial hemorrhage, midline shift, or mass effect. The normal grey–white differentiation is preserved. The ventricle and sulci are of expected size and morphology for the patient's age. Imaged paranasal sinuses and mastoid air cells are clear.
- Impression:
  - Normal CT scan of the head.

Neck CT Scan

- History:
  - Hoarseness.
- Technique:
  - CT images in the axial plane were obtained from the level of the frontal sinuses inferiorly to the thoracic inlet following the uneventful administration of intravenous contrast agent.
- Findings:
  - The spaces of the neck are normal in appearance. There are no enlarged lymph nodes, nor nodes with low-density centers. There are no abnormal areas of enhancement demonstrated.
- Impression:
  - Normal contrast-enhanced neck CT scan.

Head MR Scan

- History:
  - Headache.
- Technique:
  - Multiplanar multisequence MR images of the brain are obtained before and after intravenous administration of 20 ml of gadolinium-DTPA. Sequences obtained include: axial T1, sagittal T1, axial FLAIR, axial T2, DWI, axial/coronal T1 post-gadolinium administration. No similar prior study is available for comparison.

- Findings:
  - No signal abnormality is seen on the T1-W or T2-W images. Normal flow voids are seen in the major intracranial vessels. The ventricles and sulci are of expected size and morphology for the patient's age. There is no abnormal restriction of diffusion. Following administration of gadolinium, no abnormal enhancement is seen. The imaged paranasal sinuses and mastoid air cells are clear. Globes and orbits are unremarkable.

- Impression:
  - Normal MRI of the brain.

MRI of the Cervical Spine

- History:
  - Pain and paresthesias in left arm.

- Technique:
  - The following imaging sequences were performed: Sagittal T1-W and T2-W images from the foramen magnum to the T2 level. Axial T2-W images from the C2 level inferiorly through the T1 level.

- Findings:
  - The cervical spine is anatomic in alignment. There is no evidence of posterior disc protrusions. The spinal canal is adequately patent. No cord signal abnormalities are demonstrated.
  - Axial images at the C2–3 level: the spinal canal and neural foramina are adequately patent.
  - Axial images at the C3–4 level: the spinal canal and neural foramina are adequately patent.
  - Axial images at the C4–5 level: the spinal canal and neural foramina are adequately patent.
  - Axial images at the C5–6 level: the spinal canal and neural foramina are adequately patent.
  - Axial images at the C6–7 level: the spinal canal and neural foramina are adequately patent.
  - Axial images at the C7–T1 level: the spinal canal and neural foramina are adequately patent.

- Impression:
  - Normal cervical spine MRI.

MRI of the Lumbosacral Spine

- History:
  - Right radiculopathy.

- Technique:
  - Sagittal T1-W and T2-W images were performed from the T12 level inferiorly to the S2 level. Axial T1-W and T2-W images were performed from the L3 level through the S1 level.

- Findings:
  - The alignment of the lumbosacral spine is anatomic. There is no evidence of disc herniation. There is a normal disc hydration signal demonstrated. The conus medullaris is normal in signal intensity.
  - Axial images at the L2–3 level: the spinal canal and neural foramina are adequately patent.
  - Axial images at the L3–4 level: the spinal canal and neural foramina are adequately patent.
  - Axial images at the L4–5 level: the spinal canal and neural foramina are adequately patent.
  - Axial images at the L5–S1 level: the spinal canal and neural foramina are adequately patent.

- Impression:
  - Normal lumbosacral spine MRI.

Babygram

- History:
  - Abdominal pain.

- Findings:
  - The lungs are clear and normally inflated. The cardiothymic silhouette is within normal limits. The bowel gas pattern is unremarkable with no sign of abnormal distention or obstruction. No free air or air-fluid levels are seen on the supine view. There is no evidence of organomegaly or abnormal calcifications. No bony abnormalities are seen.

- Impression:
  - Normal babygram.

Air Enema for Intussusception Reduction

- History:
  - Suspected intussusception.

- Findings:
  - After informed consent was obtained from the patient's mother, a rubber catheter was placed in the rectum and air was gently insufflated by hand pressure. Air filled a normal colon with no intraluminal filling defect to suggest the presence of intussusception. Reflux of air into the terminal ileum and distention of small bowel was noted.

- Impression:
  - No evidence of intussusception by air enema.

Pediatric Renal and Bladder Sonography

- History:
  - Trace hydronephrosis on prenatal ultrasound scan.

- Findings:
  - The right kidney measures ... cm in length and the left kidney measures ... cm.
  - There is no evidence of hydronephrosis, hydroureter or stones. Renal echogenicity is within normal limits.
  - The filled bladder contains ... ml of urine and shows no debris or stones. Bladder wall thickness is normal. There is no post-void residual.

- Impression:
  - Normal renal and bladder ultrasound scan.

Aortogram and Bilateral Runoff

- Preprocedure diagnosis:
  - Bilateral claudication.

- Postprocedure diagnosis:
  - Status post-abdominal aortography, bilateral pelvic oblique angiography, and bilateral lower extremity runoff.

- Physicians:
  - Dr. Smith, Dr. Prodi.

- Procedures performed:
  - Right common femoral (left common femoral, left humeral) artery puncture.

- Abdominal aortography.
- Nonselective bilateral pelvic oblique angiography.
- Bilateral lower extremity runoff angiography.

- Anesthesia and medication:
  - 5 ml 1% lidocaine locally to right CFA (left CFA, left humeral artery) puncture site; intravenous Fentanyl and Versed as per usual conscious sedation protocol.

- Description of procedure:
  - Informed consent was obtained.
  - The patient was prepped and draped in the usual sterile fashion.
  - The right/left CFA (common femoral artery) was localized by palpation. 1% lidocaine solution was infiltrated subcutaneously and into the soft tissues adjacent to the right/left CFA, which in turn was entered using the Seldinger technique.
  - A guidewire was threaded to the suprarenal abdominal aorta and appropriate puncture site dilatation to 5F was achieved over the wire.
  - A 5F pigtail catheter was placed over the wire in the abdominal aorta with its tip at the level of the main renal arteries, which was confirmed with the hand injection of 5 ml contrast agent.
  - Abdominal aortography in the AP (lateral, and shallow LAO) projection was performed. The catheter was partially withdrawn to just above the aortic bifurcation and bilateral pelvic oblique angiograms were obtained. Using the station-by-station method, bilateral lower extremity runoff was then accomplished. The pigtail catheter was removed and manual pressure was applied for 15 minutes to achieve hemostasis. No significant groin hematoma was found and bilateral lower extremity pulses were unchanged as compared with preprocedure. The patient tolerated the procedure well, with no immediate complications, and was returned to the ward in good condition.

- Findings:
  - The abdominal aorta is patent and demonstrates normal caliber. The celiac artery, SMA, and IMA are patent and without significant stenoses. Right and left renal arteries are identified and are without significant disease. The bilateral common iliac, internal iliac, and external iliac arteries are patent and without significant stenoses.
  - The right PFA, SFA, popliteal artery, anterior tibial artery, tibioperoneal trunk, peroneal artery, posterior tibial artery, dorsalis pedis artery, and primary pedal arch are patent and without significant stenoses or occlusions.
  - The left PFA, SFA, popliteal artery, anterior tibial artery, tibioperoneal trunk, peroneal artery, posterior tibial artery, dorsalis pedis artery, and primary pedal arch are patent and without significant stenoses or occlusions.

- Impression:
  - Successful abdominal aortogram, bilateral pelvic angiogram, and bilateral lower extremity runoff demonstrating no significant abnormalities.

CT-Guided Abscess Drainage

- Preprocedure diagnosis:
  - Presacral abscess.

- Postprocedure diagnosis:
  - Status after successful placement of 12F catheter in presacral space.

- Physicians:
  - Dr. Walker, Dr. Ho.

- Procedures performed:
  - Limited CT scan of pelvis to localize abscess in presacral space.
  - CT-guided penetration of 19 gauge needle with aspiration of 120 ml pus.
  - Fluoroscopically guided placement of 12F drainage catheter over a wire into presacral space.
  - Injection of iodinated contrast agent through drainage catheter to confirm its position and evaluate cavity.

- Anesthesia and medication:
  - 5 ml 1% lidocaine in soft tissues overlying the target of drainage.

- Description of procedure and findings:
  - Informed consent was obtained. The patient was prepped and draped in the usual sterile fashion. A limited noncontrast CT scan of the pelvis was performed, revealing a presacral abscess. The soft tissues of the right gluteal region were infiltrated with lidocaine for local anesthesia and a 1-cm 25-gauge needle was left in place. A repeat CT scan was perfumed to confirm the position of the needle relative to the fluid collection. A 19-gauge needle was attached to a syringe and advanced parallel to the marker needle and into the fluid collection, with immediate aspiration of 120 ml pus when the needle penetrated the fluid collection. The syringe and marker needle were removed and a wire was advanced through the needle under fluoroscopic observation. The needle was removed and serial dilatation to 12F was achieved over the wire. A 12F drainage catheter was advanced over the wire into the cavity. The wire was removed, the catheter loop was secured, and the catheter position was confirmed fluoroscopically with injection of several milliliters of iodinated contrast agent. The drainage catheter was secured to the skin with a single 0 silk suture and the exit site was covered with a dry sterile dressing.

- The patient tolerated the procedure well, with no immediate complications, and was returned to the ward in good condition.
- Impression:
  - Status after successful CT and fluoroscopically guided drainage of presacral abscess.

IVC Filter Placement

- Preprocedure diagnosis:
  - Clot in the right superficial femoral vein in a 66-year-old male patient.

- Postprocedure diagnosis:
  - Status after successful placement of infrarenal IVC filter.

- Procedures performed:
  - Ultrasound-guided micropuncture of (right internal jugular, right common femoral) vein.
  - Inferior vena cavogram.
  - Fluoroscopically guided placement of IVC filter in the infrarenal IVC.

- Anesthesia and medication:
  - 5 ml 1% lidocaine at the venous puncture site.

- *Description of* procedure and findings:
  - *Informed consent was obtained. Patency of the* (right internal jugular vein, right common femoral vein) was confirmed by ultrasound. The patient was prepped and draped in the usual sterile fashion. Lidocaine was infiltrated into the soft tissues over the venous puncture site. The (right IJV, right CFV) was entered using a micropuncture technique. A 0.018-inch guidewire was threaded and appropriate dilatation to 5F was achieved over the wire. The wire was replaced with a 0.035 wire, with its tip in the IVC. A 5F pigtail catheter was placed over the wire with tip near the IVC bifurcation and the wire was removed. An inferior vena cavogram was performed to determine the level of the renal veins. The catheter was removed over the wire, progressive dilatation to 12F was achieved, and the 14F introducer sheath was placed with its tip inferior to the renal veins. The wire was removed. An IVC filter was loaded into the introducer and deployed in the infrarenal IVC under fluoroscopic observation. The introducer was removed and hemostasis was achieved with 10 minutes of manual pressure. The patient tolerated the procedure well, with no immediate complications, and was returned to the ward in stable condition.

- Impression:
  - Successful placement of IVC filter in the infrarenal IVC.

Your First Radiological Reports in English

Our advice is that you must use standard normal reports as a reference and build several "pluripathological" reports which include the most common abnormalities so that you can simply choose the sentences that fit your particular case. Once again write the sentences containing either normal findings or common pathology so that you become familiar with their spelling.

Let us have a look at this example of a "pluripathological" knee MR report which includes many usual expressions, sentences, and collocations that can help you in your first reports in English. (The following report does not intend to be a comprehensive MR knee report but a simple exercise to give you an idea of how to write your own standard reports.):

1. **No degenerative osseous changes are seen.**
   11. Gonarthrosis.

2. **Femoropatellar joint is unremarkable.**
   21. Free intraarticular fluid.
   22. No images of chondromalacia are seen.
   23. Diffuse hyperintensity on T2-W images of the hyaline cartilage of the patella consistent with grade 1 chondromalacia.
   24. Irregularity of the surface of the external aspect of the hyaline cartilage of the patella consistent with grade 2 chondromalacia.
   25. External/internal patellar subluxation.
   26. External/internal patellar luxation.
   27. Patella's retinacula without images of disruption.
   28. Internal/external retinaculum partial tear.
   29. Internal/external retinaculum complete tear.
   210. Medial/suprapatellar/infrapatellar patellar plica is unremarkable.
   211. Medial patellar plica is thickened and trapped between the patella and the femur; the finding is consistent with plica syndrome.

3. **Anterior cruciate ligament (ACL) is intact.**
   31. Partial/complete tear of the ACL.
   32. Intact ACL graft.
   33. Torn ACL graft.
   34. ACL cyst.

4. **Posterior cruciate ligament (PCL) is intact.**
   41. Partial/complete tear of the PCL.
   42. PCL cyst.

5. **Medial collateral ligament (MCL) is intact.**
   51. Distension (grade 1 lesion) of MCL.
   52. Abnormal signal intensity secondary to grade 2 lesion of MCL.
   53. Complete tear (grade 3 lesion) of MCL.

6. **Lateral collateral ligament (LCL) is intact.**
   61. Distension (grade 1 lesion) of LCL.
   62. Abnormal signal intensity secondary to grade 2 lesion of LCL.
   63. Complete tear (grade 3 lesion) of LCL.
7. **Popliteus tendon is intact.**
   71. Torn popliteus tendon.
8. **Iliotibial band is intact.**
   81. Fluid around the iliotibial (IT) band consistent with iliotibial syndrome.
9. **Menisci are unremarkable.**
   91. Grade 1 lesion of the body or anterior/posterior horn of the medial/lateral meniscus.
   92. Grade 2 lesion of the body or anterior/posterior horn of the medial/lateral meniscus.
   93. Oblique=horizontal, vertical, peripheral, radial (parrot beak) tear (grade 3 lesion) of the body or anterior/posterior horn of the internal meniscus.
   94. Bucket-handle tear of the internal meniscus.
   95. Meniscocapsular separation.
   96. Internal meniscus parameniscal cyst.
   97. External meniscus parameniscal cyst.
10. **Quadriceps tendon is unremarkable.**
    101. Partial/complete tear of the quadriceps tendon.
11. **Patellar tendon is unremarkable.**
    111. Partial tear of the proximal portion of the patellar tendon (jumper's knee).
12. **No images of bursitis are seen.**
    121. Popliteal (Baker's) cyst.
    122. Prepatellar bursitis.
    123. Pes anserinus bursitis.
    124. Semimembranous tibial collateral ligament bursitis.
    125. Tibial collateral ligament bursitis.
    126. Medial collateral ligament bursitis.
13. **No images of bone contusion are seen.**
    131. Bone contusion on the medial/lateral femoral condyle/tibial plateau.
    132. No osteochondral lesions are seen.
    133. Osteochondral lesion on the articular surface of the medial/lateral femoral condyle/tibial plateau/patella.
    134. Osteochondritis dissecans on the articular surface of the medial/lateral femoral condyle/tibial plateau/patella.
14. **No soft tissue lesions are seen.**
    141. Plantaris tendon partial/complete tear (tennis leg).

Elaborate the reports you are usually required to dictate and use them systematically.

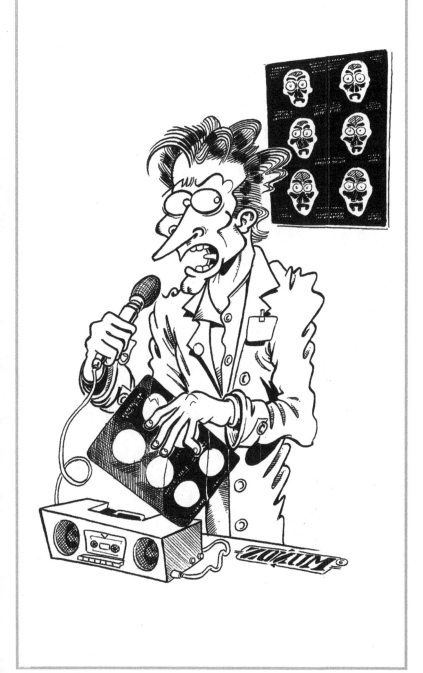

Unit XIII   Reporting in English

The scarcity of linguistic guidelines and the lack of consensus about what constitutes a good report are two of the main reasons why most residents receive little formal instruction in dictating radiological reports.

Although the elaboration of a radiological report may depend on the style, preferences, and even biases of each radiologist, a certain standard must be followed. In this unit we show some examples of the most common sentences you can use to write radiological reports. Most examples are most suitable for CT and MR imaging since these are the studies that are most commonly reported in tele-radiology.

This unit contains a short section on dictating radiological reports where tips on the dictation rhythm, usual dictation mistakes and misunderstandings, and the use of punctuation signs are given.

Usual Expressions Used in Reporting

Clinical History

- Sarcoid
  - [*say the disease*].
- Assess for, Evaluate for
  - *Assess for metastases.*
  - *Evaluate for metastases/meniscal tear.*
- Suspected
  - *Suspected pneumonia/pneumothorax/ACL tear.*
- Rule out
  - *Rule out metastases/joint effusion/fracture.*
- Status post
  - *The patient is status post left knee arthroplasty/medial meniscectomy.*

Technique

- Was/were performed
  - *Multiplanar imaging of the left knee was performed using the standard protocol.*
- Was/were obtained
  - *AP/Frontal, lateral and tangential/oblique views of the [left knee] were obtained.*

Reporting

- There is no evidence of
  - *There is no evidence of active bleeding.*
  - *There is no evidence of drainable abscess collection, glenohumeral joint effusion or osteomyelitis.*
- Suggestive of
  - *These findings are suggestive of ACL tear.*
- There is suggestion of
  - *There is suggestion of mild positive ulnar variance associated with sub-chondral cystic changes seen in the lunate.*
- Consistent with/(most) compatible with
  - *Consistent with/compatible with pneumonia/enchondroma ...*
  - *The pattern of inflammatory change is most compatible with rheumatoid arthritis.*
  - *These findings are consistent with the patient's history of spondyloepiphyseal dysplasia.*
  - *There is mild signal abnormality seen in the supraspinatus tendon at its insertion, consistent with tendinosis.*
- Is/Are unremarkable, is/are intact, appear normal, is/are normal
  - *The popliteal vessels are unremarkable.*
  - *The anterior cruciate ligament, posterior cruciate ligament, medial collateral ligament and lateral collateral ligament complex are intact.*
  - *The patellofemoral compartment appears normal.*
  - *The medial meniscus is intact.*
  - *Bone mineralization is normal.*
- To a lesser extent/degree; to a greater extent/degree
  - *Degenerative changes are seen in the PIP joint of the thumb. To a lesser degree there is mild joint space narrowing seen in the DIP joints of the 1st, 3rd, 4th, and 5th fingers.*

- There is/are, is/are present, is/are seen, is/are visualized, is/are identified
  - *There is lateral/medial subluxation of the patella.*
  - *There is focal/diffuse bone marrow edema.*
  - *There is [no] chondromalacia of the patella or osteochondral defect within the patella.*
  - *Osteophyte formation is seen in the patellofemoral compartment.*
  - *There is a physiological amount of joint fluid.*
  - *A discoid lateral meniscus is present.*
  - *No acute fracture is identified.*
  - *No focal cartilage defects are seen.*

- Within normal limits
  - *Popliteal artery and vein are within normal limits.*
  - *Marrow signal is age appropriate and within normal limits.*

- Remainder/remaining
  - *The remainder of the pelvis is unremarkable.*
  - *The remainder of the bones and cartilage spaces, including the hip, appear normal.*
  - *Remaining visualized bones are without evidence of fracture or dislocation.*

- Associated with
  - *Mild positive ulnar variance associated with chondromalacia of the lunate.*

- Right greater than left
  - *Multiple erosions throughout both hands are seen, right greater than left, consistent with given history of JRA.*

- Age appropriate
  - *Marrow signal is age appropriate and within normal limits.*

- Involving
  - *There is a tear involving the body and posterior horn of the lateral meniscus.*
  - *There is diffuse osteopenia, particularly involving the greater and lesser trochanters bilaterally, consistent with stress shielding.*

- (Most/less) likely represent
  - *There are mixed sclerotic and lucent lesions in the tips of the scapulae bilaterally with the appearance of a chondroid matrix. These findings most likely represent enchondromas. Less likely on the differential would be metastasis.*
  - *In the left hip, there is a lucency at the lateral aspect of the femoral component stem, most likely representing granulation response.*

- Seen best on/in
  - *There is elevation of the meniscus at its root attachment seen best on the coronal sequences with the avulsed fragment elevated in relation to the body of the lateral meniscus.*
  - *There is some irregularity noted of the distal fibula seen best in the oblique view.*

- Incidental note made of
  - *Incidental note made of linear low signal abnormality extending centrally into the patellofemoral joint.*

- Note is made ...
  - *Note is made of an accessory soleus muscle.*

- For further evaluation
  - *A bone scan is recommended for further evaluation.*

- Is noted
  - *Subcutaneous edema is noted along the lateral superficial soft tissues about the knee.*

- About (around)
  - *Subcutaneous edema is noted along the lateral superficial soft tissues about the knee.*
  - *There is a joint effusion about the ankle.*

- Throughout (in all parts of)
  - *Normal bone marrow signal is identified throughout the knee.*

- Show/reveal/demonstrate
  - *AP and lateral views of the left tibia and fibula reveal/show no evidence of fracture or malalignment.*
  - *Review of the bone windows demonstrates no bony abnormality.*

- Interval development
  - *Three views of the right ankle are compared with the prior study from [date] and reveal interval development of abnormal soft-tissue density overlying the right heel extending to the posterior aspect of the calcaneus which demonstrates irregularity of the cortical surface.*

Describing Different Radiological Features

- Enhancement
  - *After administration of gadolinium there is mild enhancement at ...*
  - *After administration of gadolinium no enhancement is seen at ...*
  - *No abnormal muscular edema or enhancement is seen.*

- Fracture
  - *There is a non-displaced/displaced fracture of [say the bone] with/ without intraarticular extension.*
  - *There is widening of the [say the joint] joint.*
  - *There is a fracture through the proximal lateral aspect of the [fibula ...]. The conjoined tendon is attached to the avulsed fragment.*
  - *No acute fracture or marrow edema is seen in the [distal femur, proximal tibia ...].*
  - *Standard views of the left wrist demonstrate transverse fracture with mild impaction of the distal radius. There is no definite extension to the articular surface. Remaining visualized bones are without evidence of fracture or dislocation. There is soft-tissue swelling and possible hematoma over the anterior surface of the wrist and hands.*
  - *There is an acute fracture of the lateral tibial plateau which is comminuted and extends to the articular surface. Associated edema is noted.*
  - *The left transverse process of L5 is fractured.*

- Degenerative changes
  - *Small marginal osteophytes are seen in all three compartments.*
  - *Subchondral osteophytes and sclerosis are seen in the lateral femoral trochlea.*
  - *There are well-defined erosions with sclerotic borders on both sides of the joint.*

- Soft tissue mass
  - *The right thigh shows no soft tissue or bone abnormality.*
  - *The present study shows increase in size of a lobulated mass located in the left adductor longus muscle. It presently measures 5.1×4.3 cm. Compared with the prior study in addition to the increase in size, the lesion now has a heterogeneous signal with fluid-fluid levels indicating the presence of blood products.*
  - *There is surrounding muscle edema as seen on the prior examination.*
  - *After the intravenous administration of gadolinium the lesion enhances peripherally. There is also enhancement of the adjacent muscle where edema was visualized.*
  - *The mass is again seen in proximity to the superficial femoral artery which appears preserved.*

- Elbow example (lateral epicondylitis)
  - *The medial elbow tendons are normal. Laterally, abnormal increased signal involving the common extensor tendon at its attachment to the lateral humeral epicondyle is noted. Some surrounding fluid at this site is also noted. Superficially, there is soft tissue prominence noted, accounting for the clinically palpable soft tissue "mass". Findings are most consistent with lateral epicondylitis with high-grade partial tear involving the attachment of the common extensor tendon.*

- Shoulder example
  - *There is a significant amount of fluid seen along the subdeltoid bursa with a lesser amount along the subacromial bursa. Additionally, a small heterogeneous signal lesion is seen in the subdeltoid bursa adjacent to the biceps tendon likely corresponding to the calcification seen on the prior radiograph. No glenohumeral effusion seen. No evidence of abscess formation seen. Anterior subcutaneous T2 hyperintensity likely corresponding to prior joint aspiration.*

- Plain film examples
  - *AP, lateral and sunrise views of the left knee reveal osteophyte formations, subchondral sclerosis and cartilaginous space narrowing at the patellofemoral, medial and lateral tibial femoral compartments. There is no soft tissue abnormality. AP and lateral views of the left tibia and fibula reveal no evidence of fracture or malalignment. Bone mineralization is normal.*
  - *AP and lateral views of the thoracic spine show no fracture or dislocation. The bones and cartilage spaces appear normal. No soft tissue abnormalities are seen. In these views, the right shoulder and scapula appear normal.*

- Technique
  - *AP/Frontal, lateral and tangential/oblique views of the [left knee ...] were obtained.*
  - *Comparison is made with radiographs of the same date at 18:47 hours.*
  - *No prior studies are available for comparison.*
  - *Compared with the prior study, there has been ...*

- Miscellaneous
  - *A marker is pointing to the palpable mass/DIP joint of the 2nd digit.*
  - *This is unchanged in size and appearance compared with prior plain film ... and its appearance is consistent with that of a giant bone island.*
  - *There is no evidence of fracture or dislocation.*
  - *Bony mineralization is normal.*
  - *No osteolytic or osteoblastic lesions are seen.*
  - *Two views of the right knee and two views of the right femur are submitted for evaluation without prior studies for comparison.*
  - *Comparison is made with the CT performed [date].*
  - *Note is made of a thin dark linear structure seen within the tendon sheath of the flexor digitorum longus consistent with a synechia.*
  - *Metastasis or other tumors cannot be ruled out.*
  - *There is no MRI evidence for a neoplasm or abnormal soft tissue mass.*
  - *No significant joint effusion is identified.*

Knee MR Report

- Clinical history
  - *Left knee pain, swelling, status post-skiing injury. Evaluate for meniscal tear or bone bruise. Rule out meniscal tear.*

- Protocol
  - *Multiplanar MR images of the left knee were obtained using the Standard protocol.*
  - *Multiplanar sequences were obtained of both knees with and without the intravenous administration of gadolinium, using a knee coil.*
  - *Routine MR protocol of the knee was performed.*
  - *No prior studies are available for comparison.*
  - *A comparison is made with the prior examination dated 27 November 2001.*
  - *Utilizing a dedicated coil, multiplanar sequences of the [left knee ...] were acquired without gadolinium administration.*

- Menisci
  - *A discoid lateral/medial meniscus is present.*
  - *The medial and lateral menisci are intact.*
  - *There is a (complex) tear involving the [anterior/posterior horn, body] of the lateral/medial meniscus.*

- Cruciate ligaments
  - *The posterior/anterior cruciate ligament is intact.*
  - *The anterior and posterior cruciate ligaments are intact.*
  - *There is a full-thickness tear of the ACL/PCL at its femoral/tibial insertion.*
  - *The PCL/ACL remains intact.*
  - *There is a complete tear of the anterior/posterior cruciate ligament.*

- Collateral ligaments/extensor mechanism
  - *The medial and lateral collateral ligaments are intact. The extensor mechanism is intact.*
  - *The medial and lateral collateral ligament complex and extensor mechanism are intact.*
  - *Grade 1/Grade 2 sprain of the medial/lateral collateral ligament.*
  - *The MCL/LCL is thickened but intact. The appearance of the MCL/LCL in the setting of surrounding edema is consistent with MCL/LCL sprain.*
  - *The lateral collateral ligament complex including the conjoined tendon remains intact.*

- Cartilage
  - *The lateral tibiofemoral and medial tibiofemoral compartments are normal.*
  - *There is no focal osteochondral defect.*

– There is a focal narrow area of high signal within the cartilage of the medial patellar facet consistent with a deep fissure.
– Deep fissure within the cartilage of the medial patellar facet.
– There is diffuse thinning of cartilage along the medial femoral condyle.
– No focal cartilage defect seen in the lateral compartment.
– There is mild cartilage thinning of the medial and lateral compartments.
– The articular cartilage within the knee is normal.
– There is a ... cm defect within the cartilage along the [lateral tibial plateau ...]. with approximately ... mm of depression.
– The medial tibiofemoral compartment has no focal cartilaginous defect.
– The patellofemoral compartment appears normal.

- Bones
  – Extensive bone marrow signal abnormality within the femur, tibia and fibula, sparing the epiphysis, is low on T1 and heterogeneously bright on STIR. This is consistent with the patient's history of known sickle cell anemia with early bone marrow edema.
  – There is abnormal signal within the [anterior/posterior lateral/medial tibial plateau/femoral condyle] consistent with a bone bruise.
  – No other abnormal bony findings are seen.
  – There is no bone marrow edema.
  – Normal bone marrow signal is identified throughout the knee.

- Other (miscellaneous)
  – There is no significant joint effusion.
  – There is a large joint effusion.
  – There is a mild/moderate [say the joint] joint effusion.
  – There is a physiological amount of joint fluid.
  – There are no muscle abnormalities/soft tissue edema.
  – Soft tissue swelling is present around the site of injury.
  – A small popliteal cyst is identified.
  – No popliteal cyst is identified.
  – Prepatellar subcutaneous edema.
  – There is no evidence of acute fracture or dislocation.
  – There is no significant joint space narrowing.
  – Early tricompartmental osteoarthritic changes.
  – There is focal high signal demonstrated within the patellar tendon near its insertion.
  – There is no chondromalacia of the patella or osteochondral defect within the patella.
  – There is minimal lateral subluxation of the patella.
  – There is lateral subluxation of the patella.
  – Osteophyte formation is seen in the patellofemoral compartment/medial tibiofemoral compartment/lateral tibiofemoral compartment.

- *[say the muscle] is surrounded by fluid and demonstrates increased signal within the substance of the tendon. Findings are consistent with extensive partial tear.*
- *Fluid is present within the tendon sheath of [say the muscle], consistent with tenosynovitis*

- Recommendations
  - *Six-week MR follow-up to assess for healing is appropriate if clinically indicated.*
  - *Further evaluation by pelvic sonography or MRI is recommended.*
  - *Further evaluation with arthroscopy may be of further diagnostic value.*
  - *Findings were called in to the orthopedic resident/attending at the time of dictation.*
  - *This result was paged to beeper number 111111 at the time of interpretation.*
  - *5 mm nodular opacity in the right lower lobe is indeterminate. If a prior study is available, it may be used to establish stability. Alternatively, a repeat study may be obtained in ... months.*
  - *The 4 mm right adrenal nodule has signal characteristics compatible with an adenoma. No further imaging is recommended unless the patient's clinical status changes.*
  - *Short segment inflammation of the descending colon may be a manifestation of diverticulitis but the asymmetric wall thickening is concerning. Further study should be considered once the acute inflammation has resolved to exclude an underlying process.*
  - *Incidentally seen right adnexal cystic mass is not adequately evaluated on CT. A pelvic ultrasound scan would be the next study of choice.*

- CT/MR limitations
  - *Image quality is degraded by motion.*
  - *Images of the pelvis are limited by streak artifact from the right hip prosthesis.*
  - *Degree of contrast opacification of the pulmonary artery is not adequate to exclude a pulmonary embolus.*
  - *Absence of intravenous contrast lowers the sensitivity of the study for detection of vascular lesions.*
  - *Presence of intravenous contrast lowers sensitivity of the study for detection of small renal stones.*

Dictating a Radiological Report

Appropriate dictating either to a secretary or to a speech recognition device results in faster report turnaround and reduces waiting times for patients and referring physicians.

Many radiologists are convinced that dictating quickly serves to expedite the work and is a reflection of their knowledge of radiology. Accordingly, residents are perceived as slow dictators, a notion supported in part by the their lack of experience and emerging knowledge base. In our opinion, both ideas are incomplete. The sensation of having done the work is false unless the dictation is complete and correct. Hence, clear and error-free dictation is paramount.

The first piece of advice to dictate reports is: talk to your secretary! (or, in this era of speech recognition systems, train your speech recognition software!). Tell your secretary to make a list of his/her mistakes and think about how many of them could have been avoided with better dictation.

When I was a research fellow at Brigham and Women's Hospital in Boston I wondered why the attending radiologist cleared his throat at the end of certain reports. As time went by I realized that this experienced and "fast-dictating" radiologist only cleared his throat at the end of the reports of patients suffering from ... *hiatal hernia*! The way in which he said "hiatal hernia" was absolutely impossible to understand not only by me but by every foreign resident rotating in this section at that time. From then on that extraordinarily fast "hiatal hernia" comes to my mind whenever I have to clear my throat giving a lecture.

Standard Dictation

1. "This is Dr. ... dictating" <your name>
2. "Dictating with" <attending's name> (only if you are a resident or fellow)
3. "Patient" <patient's name>, "accession number" <accession no. of the study>
4. "Chest PA and lateral, KUB, MR with and without contrast ..." <study type>
5. "Dated" <date and time of study>
6. "Compared with" <comparison studies, if available>
7. "Clinical history:" <given history>
8. *Optional*: "Technique" <describe the technique> (only dictated for CT scans, fluoro studies, HSGs and any procedure where technique is significant).
9. "Findings:" <any findings that are appropriate>

10. "Impression:" <conclude with an impression, usually in numbered bullet format>
11. "End of dictation"

Dictation Example

This is Dr. Smith dictating with Dr. Pole.
  Patient Joseph Taylor, Accession number 87654.
  Study is chest PA and lateral dated May 21, 04 compared with chest PA from August 28, 03 at 08:00.
  Clinical history <colon> cough and fever <period> <paragraph>
  Findings <colon> two views of the chest demonstrate dense medial lobe consolidation obscuring the right heart border as well as part of the right hemidiaphragm <comma> with interval worsening of the same findings from prior study <period> Cardiac size is again increased and unchanged <period> Prior healed rib fractures are again noted on the right side <period> <paragraph>
  Impression <colon> Number one <comma> medial lobe pneumonia <comma> worsening as compared with yesterday's film <period> Number two <comma> increased heart size <period> End of dictation.

Next patient ...
  ...
End of dictation. Thanks.

Dictating Puntuation Marks, Eponyms, Acronyms and Abbreviations

.	Period (full-stop)
:	Colon
;	Semicolon
,	Comma
(	Open parenthesis
)	Close parenthesis
5F	F in capital letters
FLAIR	In capital letters
May-Turner	Both beginning with capital letters and separated by a hyphen
-	Hyphen
?	Interrogation mark

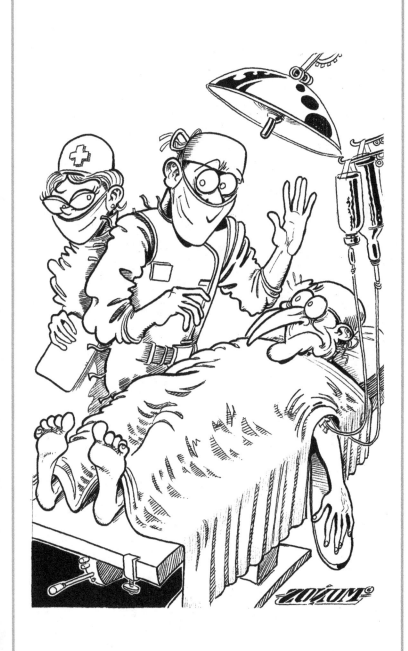

Unit XIV   Interventional Radiology

Introduction

IR suites are real-time decision-making environments in which lack of fluency can be troublesome not only for the non-native English-speaking radiologist but for anybody else in the laboratory, the patient included. This is the reason why we have dedicated a complete unit to interventional radiology.

When you enter an IR suite your listening skills are much more important than your fluency; nobody is expecting you to say too much but everybody takes for granted that you understand them, and that is not always true. You will find no difficulty when the conversation is on the pathology itself; in the first few days many jargon terms, acronyms, and abbreviations can be tricky but, with a bit of help, you will soon feel reasonably confident.

Do you know, for example, what a SOAP note is? If you haven't worked in an American hospital, probably not. SOAP stands for (Subjective comments on the patient, Objective findings, Assessment, and Plan) and SOAP note refers to the standard follow-up chart entries.

One of the main problems of non-native English-speaking interventional radiologists working in English-speaking IR suites is the lack of knowledge of basic vocabulary, jargon terminology, acronyms, abbreviations, and set phrases.

Let us begin with this simple conversation that may have happened hundreds of times in IR suites. Familiarity with conversations such as the following will help in our first days in an English-speaking IR suite.

- Radiologist getting ready for case, speaking to IR technologist: "I'll be in as soon as I get the cap, facemask, and booties on."
- IR technologist: "I'll have your gown ready for you. What size gloves do you take?"
- Radiologist: "I usually take 8's but I'm going to double-glove for this case, so I'll take 8 under and 8 1/2 on top. Thanks."

The first thing a foreigner notices in an IR suite is that he/she is not familiar with terminology regarding garments since he/she has not asked for garments in English before and because virtually nothing has been written on booties, masks, caps, gowns, etc.

In the following pages we will go over several sentences typical of an IR suite. Those who have not worked in an IR suite abroad and are not going to do so in the future may not see the point in reviewing so many easy set phrases; these sentences are indeed quite easy to understand for an interventional radiologist independently of his English level.

Our advice is try to read them aloud. By doing this not-that-simple exercise you will immediately notice that you may not be confident in reading aloud and pronouncing correctly some of the sentences you used to despise as simple. The best way to become familiar with the listening, pronunciation, and spelling of these sentences is to write them down and read them aloud.

When, during your first days in a foreign IR suite, you hear some of these sentences uttered by native speakers you will realize how important it was to have heard the sentences before, and you should already have practiced the first sentences you have to say yourself.

Garments

Tools and devices are usually well known by foreign radiologists since they have read about them in the literature. Garments are a different issue. Since garment terminology is so engrained in the core of the subspecialty, it is quite difficult to find written garment names; no article is going to say a word on scrubs, booties, masks, lead aprons, radiation badges ...

The most common formula to ask for anything in this environment is:

- Can I have ...?

Everyone who has rotated in an English-speaking IR suite has felt the need to ask for garments:

- Where are the lead aprons?
- Do we have lead aprons?
- This lead apron is too small. Can I have a larger one?
- Can I have a face mask?
- Could you give me a hood?
- Can you tell me know where the shoe covers are.
- I'll need a pair of lead gloves.
- What size gloves do you take? Eight.
- I'm going to double-glove for this case.
- I'll take 8 under and 8 ½ on top.
- My scrubs top is soaked. I need to change it.
- There is a blood stain on my scrubs pants (*UK* trousers).

- I left my radiation badge in my locker.

Look at the schematic representation on the following page in which we have included some of the most common IR garments.

Tools and Devices

Once you are properly dressed, you will have to ask for tools and devices. Since most tools and devices are known beforehand, we give you a few examples of usual requests and common formulas to ask for guides, stents, catheters ...:

- Can I have a 0.035 guidewire?
- Can I have a hydrophilic guidewire?
- Can I have a 5F introducer?
- Can I have a 16 G needle?
- Give me a 10F nephrostomy tube, please.
- Give me an angled Amplatz guidewire, please.
- I'd rather use a pig-tail catheter.
- The foreign body seems to have a free end; I'll use an Amplatz goose neck snare.
- Can I have a torque vise?
- Can I have a stiffer guidewire, please?

Talking to the Patient

"Don't breathe don't move" is probably the commonest command in an IR suite.

- Keep still.
- Don't breathe don't move.
- Push as if you were going to have a bowel movement (Valsalva maneuver).
- Take a deep breath and bear down as if you are going to have a bowel movement (Valsalva maneuver).
- Let me know if this hurts (to check if the local anesthetic is working properly).
- Let me know if this stings (to check if the concentration of the local anesthetic in sodium bicarbonate is adequate).
- Do you feel a warm sensation during injection? (to check if the concentration of local anesthetic in sodium bicarbonate is adequate).
- You will feel a burning sensation in your stomach during injection of the contrast material. It's nothing to worry about.

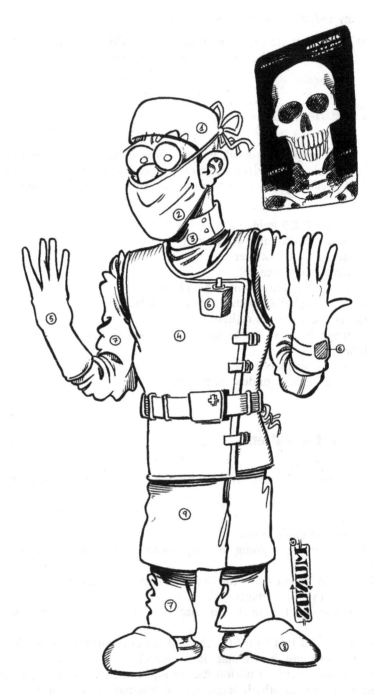

1. Cap, 2. Mask, 3. Thyroid shield, 4. Lead Apron, 5. Gloves, 6. Radiation badge, 7. Scrubs, 8. Clogs, 9. Gown

- Breathe in deeply and hold your breath.
- Breathe in deeply.
- Breath out deeply and hold your breath.

Talking to the Patient's Family

Before the Procedure

- Your father/husband/mother/wife/son/daughter is about to undergo an interventional radiology procedure (arteriography, PTA ...). It will take approximately ... minutes. The procedure does not need a general anesthetic, only local anesthesia, so your father (etc.) will remain conscious. I will let you know how the procedure went as soon as we finish.

After the Procedure

Good News

- Everything has gone fine from a technical point of view; we will look carefully at the images and the report will be sent to your father's (etc.) referring physician. In a few minutes you will see your father (etc.). He is doing fine. Please make sure he does not move his right leg for 24 hours.

Bad News

- I am afraid your father's condition is critical. He will be transferred to the ICU.
- Unfortunately, we have not been able to cross the stenosis so the patient will be transferred to the Department of Vascular Surgery where he will be operated on on an elective basis.
- There has been a serious complication. Your father is being transferred to the operating room where he will be operated on now. We (the surgeon and myself) will inform you of the situation as soon as the operation is finished.

Teaching Residents

These are some of the most common commands given in IR suites:
- Prep the patient.
- Drape the patient.
- Make sure that the patient's groin has been shaved, scrubbed and draped.
- Has the puncture site been scrubbed?
- Locate the right common femoral artery (RCFA) by palpation.
- Locate the left humeral artery by palpation.
- Puncture the artery.
- Do not force the wire.
- Inject local anesthetic as deeply as possible and don't forget to aspirate before injecting.
- Tape the lower abdominal pannus back away from the groin.
- Nick the skin with a small blade.
- Use a hemostat to fluoroscopically check the proper position of the intended entry site.
- The skin entry must be over the lower femoral head and the puncture site over the medial third of the femoral head.
- Advance the needle in a single forward thrust.
- Advance the needle by about 2–3 cm.
- Remove the stylet.
- Retract the needle slowly.
- Gently retract the syringe while keeping the position of the needle firmly fixed.
- Have you flushed the cath (catheter)?
- Have you checked for free backflow?
- Don't lose the wire.
- Hold the wire.
- Wipe the guidewire.
- Manipulate gently.
- Don't forget that the catheter tip migrates cephalad 2–3 cm after upright positioning.
- Once the dilator is introduced over the wire, exchange it for the pigtail catheter.
- Avoid axillary artery puncture because of the proximity to the brachial plexus.
- The stent is not patent.
- The ureter has been perforated.
- There is a clot in the renal pelvis.
- Remove the nephrostomy tube over the wire.
- The initial stent positioning was not appropriate.
- The stent sizing is appropriate.
- Exchange the micropuncture dilator for a peel-away sheath.

- The peel-away sheath is kinked at a sharp turn.
- Have you aspirated both lumens?
- Is there free blood return?
- Peel away the sheath.
- Introduce the catheter over the wire.
- Do not persevere with catheter manipulation.
- We could not cross the lesion.
- The coil is misplaced.
- The coil has migrated into the central venous circulation. Give me a snare device.
- Don't worry. Venous perforations are usually self-limiting.
- Tunneled catheters may have staggered or aligned tips.
- If there is no pyonephrosis, use an 8F nephrostomy tube.
- Dilate the tract up to the required French size.
- Avoid puncturing extrahepatic ducts.
- After crossing the stenosis, give 2500 IU of heparin IA.
- Size the balloon diameter equal to the adjacent normal vessel measured on cut-film arteriography.
- Cross the stenosis gently.
- Extra care must be taken with hydrophilic Glidewire to avoid dissection.
- Retract the balloon-catheter leaving the guidewire across the lesion.
- Keep the balloon deflated by suctioning with a large-bore syringe.

Talking to Nurses

- May I have my gown tied?
- Would you tie my gown?
- Tie me up, please.
- Dance with me (informal way of asking to have your gown tied).
- I'll go scrub in a minute.
- Give Dr. Ross a pair of shoe covers.
- Give Dr. Ross a thyroid shield.
- Give Dr. Ross a lead apron.
- Mary, I forgot my thyroid shield. Could you put one on me?
- Is the patient monitored yet?
- Dr. Cole, there is a phone call for you. It's Dr. Viamonte. Tell him I'll call back later; I can't break scrub now.
- May I have another pair of gloves, please?
- May I have a pair of lead gloves?
- We've had a complication. Page the thoracic surgeon.

Talking to Technologists

- Can I have this image magnified, please?
- Could you please collimate the image to minimize my hand exposure?
- An LPO 45 degrees, please.
- Right posterior oblique 45 degrees (side of interest down).
- Film at 4 to 6 frames per second during suspended respiration in antero-posterior DSA.
- Road mapping, please.

The IR's Angiographic Equipment

- The *generator* provides the electrical energy from which X-rays are generated and contains the circuitry needed to provide a controlled and stable radiation output. The mid- to high-frequency inverter is the most popular generator design.
- The *X-ray tube* is made of a tungsten filament cathode and a spinning anode disk with a tungsten surface. Electrons go from the cathode to the anode where they are stopped by its tungsten surface.
- The *image intensifier (II)* converts the X-ray pattern that penetrates the patient to an intensified image. Its fields of view range from 4 to 16 inches depending on the magnification factor.
- The *patient table* is usually made of carbon fiber to provide enough strength to support an adult patient while minimizing the attenuation of X-rays.
- The *gantry stand* contains both the X-ray tube housing with collimator and the image intensifier/imaging chain.
- High refresh-rate *TV monitors* are used to reduce flickering of the image created within the digital TV camera.
- *Contrast injectors* allow the adjustment of injection volume, peak injection rate, and acceleration to peak rate. *Contrast injector arms* can be ceiling-suspended or mounted on the table. The *injector control unit* can be on a pedestal in the procedure room or rack-mounted in the *control area*.

Some Common "On Call" Orders for Nurse Units

These are some of the commonest orders for nursing IR units. Non-native English-speaking interventional radiologists must be familiar with them in order to be able to write them down on the chart.

Patient Preparation

- Premedicate with diazepam (Valium) 10 mg PO (oral intake) given on-call to angiography (optional). Reduce dose for elderly and pediatric patients.
- Obtain informed consent.
- Patients must void urine before leaving the ward for the angiography suite.
- Transfer the patient to the angiography suite with his/her identification plate, chart, and latest laboratory reports on chart.
- The front cover of the chart should list all precautionary measures needed to protect the patient (especially if immunocompromised) and personnel (who may come into contact with patients with infectious diseases).
- Clear fluids only after midnight (for morning appointment).
- Clear fluids only after breakfast (for afternoon appointment).
- Insert Foley catheter.
- Vigorous hydration (NSS at 125 ml/h).
- Prophylactic antibiotics IV.
- Instruct patient to use PCA pump.
- Laboratory check: Hgb/Hct, platelet count, PT/PTT, BUN, and Cr.
- Establish a peripheral IV.

Postprocedure Management

- Bed rest for 6 to 8 hours, with puncture site evaluation.
- Vigorous hydration (NSS 3 l/34 h) until oral intake is adequate.
- Stop analgesics and remove Foley catheter 24 hours after the procedure.
- Monitor patient in the recovery room for 6 hours prior to discharge.
- IV narcotics (prn).
- Forward-flush the drainage catheter with normal saline every 48 hours.
- Change the dressing around the drainage catheter every 48 hours.
- Leave the catheter to gravity drainage without flushing.
- Remove catheter when there is drainage of less than 20 ml/day and vital signs return to normal.
- Follow-up ultrasound scan in 24 h.

IR Chart Entries

Standard Format

An example of a daily chart entry following uterine artery embolization (UAE) would be a SOAP note (Subjective comments, Objective findings, Assessment, Plan), as follows:

IR   PN-R3[1]
S[2]:   Pt without complaints. No nausea or pain.
O[3]:   T (max) 37.2, 82 bpm, BP: 122/78, u.o = x ml/hour
      Pt in NAD
      Chest: CTA b
      Abdo: benign, S NT, NAD
      Groin: No hematoma. Dressing c/d/i
      Ext: Warm 2+ DP, 2+ PT. Neuro sensation intact.
A/P[4]: Post UAE day 1
      1. Pt doing well post UAE. Pain well controlled.
      2. Planning d/c to home this morning.

---

[1] The first line denotes the service authoring the note and the person writing the note. In this example, "IR PN-R3" indicates that interventional radiology is the service authoring the progress note (PN). "R3" refers to the person writing the note. Typically, R means "resident" followed by the training year (3). Attending physicians will usually write "Staff".
[2] "S" is a summary of the patient's subjective comments.
[3] "O" is a summary of objective findings (including vital signs and urine/drain output) and physical examination (NAD no acute distress; CTA b clear to auscultation bilaterally; S NT soft, nontender; NAD normal active bowel sounds; c/d/i clean dry intact, DP dorsalis pedis artery; PT posterior tibial artery).
[4] "A/P" is a summary of the assessment and plan (d/c discharge).

Progress Note

While in-house, patients are followed at least daily. Daily progress notes (PN) follow the same format. Many in-house patients, particularly unit patients, have complex issues. While the IR service needs to be aware of all issues, the progress note is focused on the issues that directly impact our care.

IR   PN-R3
S: Pt intubated and sedated.
O: T 36.2–38.4 (presently 37.0), HR 78–102 (presently 86), BP 112–132/ 72–88 (presently 122/82), u.o = x ml/hour, percutaneous cholecystostomy output: xx ml/12 hours
Pt   intubated
      Percutaneous cholecystostomy site c/d/i. Dark green output (volumes as above).
      Abdomen: S NT. Diminished bowel sounds.
      Intraprocedure cultures pending.
A/P: Post Perc Chole day 2.
      1. Drainage catheter functioning without difficulty. Continue current care.
      2. Will continue to follow daily. Please page $xxxx$ if any questions arise.

IR Procedure Note

Standard Format
IR procedure note: ____

Date/Time: ____

Inpatient/Outpatient: ____

History/Indications: ____

Consent: ____ (from patient or from appropriate family member if patient unable to consent)

Radiologist: ____

Guidance modality: ____ (CT/US/fluoroscopy/MR)

Medications given: ____ (includes dose)

Needles/Catheters/Device used: ____ (includes device number)

Findings: ____

Specimen sent: ____

Complication: ____ (includes steps taken, management and/or person contacted to assist in management)

Disposition: ____ (to floor/ICU or holding followed by home if outpatient procedure)

Example 1

IR procedure note: CT guided drainage catheter placement

Date/Time: March 3, 2005

Inpatient/Outpatient: Inpatient 6D

History/Indications: 32 y.o. woman involved in MVC with LUQ intraabdominal abscess post splenectomy.

Consent: Written, informed consent obtained from patient.

Radiologist: Dr. Smith

Guidance modality: CT

Medications given: Versed 2 mg, Fentanyl 200 mcg

Needles/Catheters/Device used: 22 gauge × 10 cm needle, 14 French flexima (serial no. 123456)

Findings: Thick-walled low-density, collection in LUQ contains thick, dark-brown fluid

Specimen sent: 10 ml of dark brown fluid for GS and culture. Total 150 ml aspirated

Complication: Trace left pneumothorax. Patient remained hemodynamically stable through the procedure. 4 hours postprocedure CXR showed no PTX. Primary physician, Dr. Jones, informed of trace PTX. Plan made for close observation with repeat CXR if clinical symptoms develop.

Disposition: To floor 6D

Example 2

IR procedure note: Right IJ (internal jugular) HD (hemodialysis) catheter placement

Date/Time: March 4, 2005

Inpatient/Outpatient: Outpatient

History/Indications: 63 y.o. male with h/o DM and ESRD in need of venous access for hemodialysis.

Consent: Informed, written consent obtained from patient.

Radiologist: Dr. Smith

Guidance modality: Fluoroscopy, imaging time < 60 sec

Medications given: Fentanyl *xx* mcg, Versed *xx* mg

Needles/Catheters/Device used: MedComp Serial no. 123456

Findings: HD catheter placed via right IJ, tunneled to right anterior chest wall. Catheter tip is in mid RA. No kink along catheter course. No pneumothorax on fluoroscopy. All lumens draw blood back briskly and were terminally flushed with *xxx* U/cc of heparin.

Specimen sent: None

Complication: None

Disposition: To dialysis

Example 3
IR procedure note: Right percutaneous renal biopsy

Date/Time: March 2, 2005

Inpatient/Outpatient: Inpatient 5D

History/Indications: 54 y.o. male s/p left nephrectomy in 1997 for RCC. Newly diagnosed lung adenoCA. New right renal mass.

Consent: Informed written consent obtained from patient.

Radiologist: Dr. Smith

Guidance modality: CT

Medications given: Fentanyl *xx* mcg, Versed *xx* mg

Needles/Catheters/Device used: ... (includes device number)

Findings: ...

Specimen sent: Three samples reviewed by cytopathologist at time of biopsy.

Complication: Trace right subcapsular hematoma. Patient remained hemodynamically stable through the procedure. Primary physician, Dr. Jones, informed of right renal subcapsular hematoma. Plan made for close observation with hematocrit check/repeat CT if clinical symptoms develop.

Disposition: To floor 5C

Contrast Reactions

For contrast reactions, a form rather than chart entry is used. The information is similar and includes:

- Type and volume of contrast given
- Type and severity of reaction
- Action taken
- Future recommendation

If the form were to be written, an example would be:

Date/Time: ...
Pt Smith (MR no. 123456) developed a mild facial rash following the administration of 100 ml Ultravist 300. Patient remained hemodynamically stable and had no dyspnea. Given the mild reaction, no pharmaceutical action was taken. Patient was kept in observation for one hour, during which the rash resolved with no residual symptoms. Patient was asymptomatic at time of discharge to home. ER warning was given and contact pager of the radiologist on call provided. Patient also provided with Contrast Reaction Card for future reference. Entry of event made into medical record. Patient instructed that subsequent studies should (a) be done without contrast agent, (b) be done with proper premedication, or (c) be done using alternative modality requiring no Ultravist. Risks and benefits of study should be discussed with referring physician and radiologist at time of study.

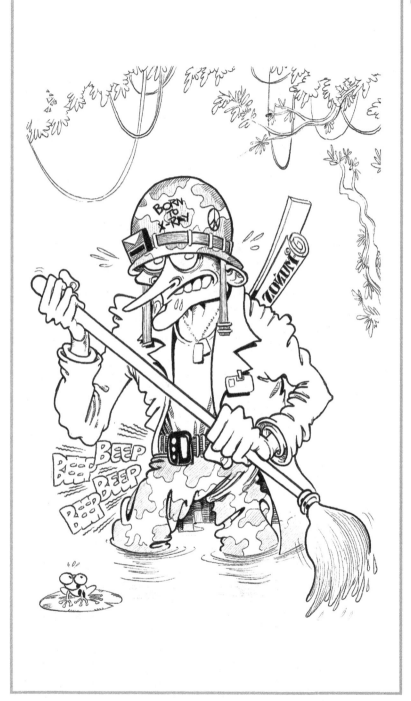

Unit XV   On Call

In this unit we review some conversations which might take place during clinical duties. Calls are a dreadful conversational scenario for beginners since it is on calls where more real-time decision-making is required and radiological English is particularly full of acronyms, abbreviations, and radiological jargon.

If you ask an American citizen, lay in medicine, what we mean by POD and CAC, take for granted that he will not say "postoperative day" and "clear all corridors", respectively. Therefore, it is an irrefutable fact that both medical and radiological English are a universe of their own, and this is even more true when we talk about calls.

We have tried to compile as many "call terms, sentences, and collocations" as possible in just a few conversations. These sentences do not need translation or any further comments and any intermediate level English-speaking radiologist can understand them easily provided they are within the appropriate context. Read the sentences aloud and do not let them catch you off guard.

Common On-Call Sentences

- A pager goes off.
- The neuroradiologist is Q4 or Q5.
- In your next golden weekend ...
- Post-call days.
- I've just reviewed your patient's MR, and wanted to discuss the findings with you.
- I would like to obtain more information on her presentation and past surgical history.
- Thank you for contacting me regarding Mrs. McHugh's CT.
- There has been no significant interval change in the appearance of ...
- I concur with the previous report.
- The next study of choice would be ...
- ER physician.
- To order a brain MR ...
- Diagnosed with ...
- Admitted for abdominal pain.

- Admitted for oncologic work up.
- Is Mrs. Smith having neurological symptoms?
- Is the brain MR for staging?
- To obtain it as a "next available" study ...
- It is not emergent.
- I'll contact the technologist.
- Resident finishing call.
- Resident coming on call.
- There are two studies pending.
- POD 10.
- Patient's medical record number #####.
- In the ICU on D10.
- The contact person for the patient is Dr. Roos.
- Her pager number is #####.
- The technologist has called for the patient.
- Transport is on the way.
- I'll follow up on these studies.
- To page the referring physician ...
- I'm the radiologist on call.
- I want to inform you about the findings.
- There is a mass in the liver.
- Paged by clinical service.
- I am returning a page. How can I help you?
- My pager is not working properly. May I have some fresh batteries?
- Is the patient under contact precautions?
- Is the patient intubated?
- Can the patient be repositioned in the left lateral decubitus position?
- I will get some extra help to move the patient.
- I will set up the ultrasound machine.
- Fiona was signing out to Amy.
- There are just a couple of brain CTs pending.
- DNR patient (baby).
- I'm on again tonight.
- I get the weekend off.
- I'll be post-call on Tuesday and Friday.
- From then on, it's "only" every third for the rest of the month.
- I got only one hit.
- I am scheduled to be on with ...
- I've woken up from my pre-call sleep.
- "Call a code!"
- CAC in the emergency room.
- It seems like every walk-in needs a brain CT.
- That make me suspicious of ...
- The IV (line) has fallen out.
- We must replace the IV line.
- Everybody was either pre-call or post-call.

On-Call Conversations

A pager goes off. A radiologist, a cardiologist, and an orthopedic surgeon are having dinner at the hospital cafeteria:
- "Whose beeper (pager) *is going off?*"
- "It has to be mine; the CT technologist must have finished the brain CT I was expecting," says the radiologist, producing his pager from his lab coat right pocket.

- "Are you Q4 or Q5?"
- "I am Q4."

- "Where are you going on your next *golden weekend*, Peter?"
- "I'm go to Spain."

- "What are the toughest days for a radiology resident, Sam?"
- "*Post-call* days are probably the toughest for a resident."

- *Radiologist:* "Good morning Dr. Walker. *I just reviewed your patient's MR, and wanted to discuss the findings with you ...*"

- *Radiologist:* "Good morning Dr. Lee. I am reviewing Mrs. Carter's abdominal US and *would like to obtain more information on her presentation and past surgical history ...*"

- *Radiologist:* "Dr Clark, *thank you for contacting me regarding Mrs. McHugh's CT.* I received her prior studies from John Hopkin's Hospital and have been able to compare them with our most recent studies. *There has been no significant interval change in the appearance of* the 4 cm liver lesion in segment VIII. *I concur with the previous report:* it could be an FNH (focal nodular hyperplasia)."

- *Radiologist:* "If the lesion in the right temporal lobe is the area of concern, *the next study of choice would be* an enhanced brain MR."

Radiology resident on call in ER (Emergency Room). Radiologist's *pager goes off.* Conversation with *ER physician* in the emergency room (ER) at 3 a.m.:
- *ER physician:* "Hello, I would like *to order a brain MR* and CT of the abdomen and pelvis for Mrs. Smith (patient). She was recently *diagnosed with* lung cancer and is *being admitted for abdominal pain* and further oncologic workup."
- *Radiologist:* "*Is Mrs. Smith having neurologic symptoms* or is the brain MR for staging?"
- *ER physician:* "For staging."
- *Radiologist:* "If patient is having no neurologic symptoms and the brain MR is requested for staging only, it is reasonable to obtain it as a '*next available*' study, since it is not *emergent*. The CT of the abdomen and

pelvis is appropriate, given patient's symptoms and will be done emergently. *I will contact the CT technologist.*"

Radiology resident *finishing call,* speaking to resident *coming on call:*
- *Radiologist 1:* "There are two *studies pending.* The first is a CT of the abdomen and pelvis on a *post op patient,* Mr. Johnson, who is *POD 10* from a gastrectomy, with persistent fevers and elevated white count. The patient's *medical record number* is #####. He is located *in the ICU on 10D.* The *contact person for the patient is Dr. Jones* (the surgery resident). *His pager number is #####;. The second is patient is Mrs. Simpson. The technologist has already been contacted and has called for the patients. Transport is on the way.*"
- *Radiologist 2:* "Thanks. *I'll follow up on these studies* and contact Dr. Jones with the results."
- *Radiologist 2* (upon review of CT, radiologist *has paged the referring physician*): "Dr. Jones, this is Dr. Miller, *I am the radiologist on call.* Thank you for calling back. I have reviewed Mr. Johnson's CT and wanted *to inform you of the findings. There is a mass in the liver ...*"

Radiology resident on call, *paged by clinical service:*
- *Radiologist:* "This is Dr. Miller. I am the radiologist on call. *I am returning a page. How can I help you?*"

- *Technologist:* "Dr. Petit, you didn't return a page from the cardiologist."
- *Radiologist:* "I haven't been paged in the last couple of hours."
- *Technologist:* "Is your pager working properly?"
- *Radiologist:* "I'm afraid it's *not working properly. Do you have some fresh batteries?*"

Doing an ultrasound examination at the ICU:
- *Radiologist* (speaking to ICU nurse): "Good afternoon, I am Dr. Miller. I am here to do Mrs. Smith's (patient) abdominal ultrasound. *Is the patient under contact precautions?*"
- *Nurse:* "Yes, patient is MRSA. The yellow contact gowns and gloves are in the drawer by the entrance."
- *Radiologist: "Is the patient intubated? Can the patient be repositioned in the left lateral decubitus position?"*
- *Nurse:* "Yes, patient is intubated but can be turned about 30 degrees. *I will get some extra help to move the patient.*"
- *Radiologist:* "Thank you. *I will set up the ultrasound machine* in the meantime."

- At about eight o'clock *Fiona was signing out to Amy* in the nurse's station. "*There are just a couple of brain CTs pending*; it's been kind of quiet."

- "The brain CT was not ordered because the patient was a *DNR baby*" (DNR stands for "do not resuscitate". DNR orders are written after careful consultation with all parties involved in the patient's care, including the child's parents.)

- "I was on call the night before last and *I'm on again tonight.* I'm doing an every other night, which is fine, because *I get the weekend off.*"
- "I am on on Monday and again on Wednesday so *I'll be post-call on Tuesday and Thursday* but *from then on it's "only" every third for the rest of the month.*"
- "How was your call, Sam?"
- "Not bad at all. I had a really easy night; *I got only one hit.*"
- "*I am scheduled to be on with* really nice attendings during my next three calls."
- "For some reason *I've woken up from my pre-call sleep.* I can't help thinking about my presentation on alveolar proteinosis."
- "*Call a code!* When I entered the room everybody was starting to position the patient to start CPR."
- "Attention, attention: *CAC* (clear all corridors) *in the emergency room.*"
- "Another brain CT? I can't believe it. *It seems like every walk-in* (every patient who comes to the emergency room) *needs a brain CT.*"
- "I just reviewed the X-rays and I see multiple fractures *that make me suspect* child abuse."
- "*The IV line has fallen out.* I'm afraid *we must replace it.*"
- "No radiology resident came to the party. *Everybody was either pre-call or post-call.*"

Additional Call Terms

- *Pre-call/post-call*: Day preceding or following call.
- "Q": Denotes frequency of call. For example, "I am Q4" means that call is taken every 4 days.
- *Golden weekend*: Weekend uninterrupted by call. For example, on a Q4 call schedule, a golden weekend is flanked by a Thursday and Monday call.
- *Home call*: Call taken from home where issues resolvable by phone are done so may require returning to the hospital for issues that require personal presence.
- *In-house call*: Person on call stays in the hospital for the duration of call.
- *Night float*: System of call where night coverage is assigned for several days in a row (usually on a weekly basis). The person on call works at night and is free of day-time responsibilities.

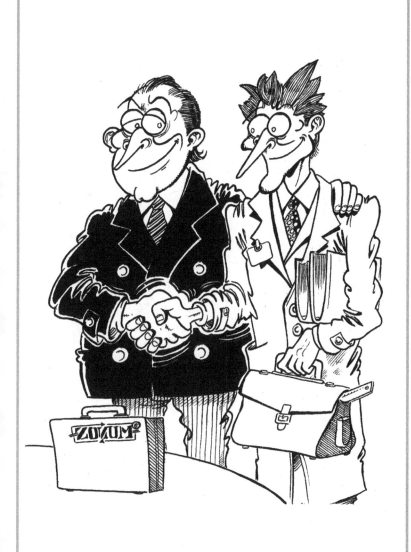

Unit XVI   Radiological Management

Diagnostic imaging represents a significant percentage of the average hospital's revenue and often an even greater percentage of the organization's contribution margin. However, improving services has turned harder in an environment of increasing competition.

Today's radiology management includes several areas of responsibility. The main areas are:

- Operations improvement
- Hospital relations
- Business planning
- Staffing
- New tool selection and implementation
- Marketing planning
- Profitability assurance
- Quality control
- Budgeting
- Patient satisfaction
- Safety surveillance

A radiology manager may be defined as a well-rounded, versatile, technically proficient, business-savvy, customer service-oriented professional with multiple years of experience, professional certifications and higher degrees employed to manage a radiology department ... seven days a week for a minimum wage.

The radiology manager has responsibility for all the above areas listed above and issues related to them. His/her focus and ultimate goal is to assure the continuous improvement of the radiology department. The radiology manager also dictates policies that aim to achieve these goals and create the necessary structure to implement and fulfil the mission of the department.

Commonly Used Phrases

- We can't hire another CT technologist, ... sorry, your extended schedule has to wait (Hospital VP for ancillary).
- What do you mean by saying that your productivity is only 30% of SCARD mean? (Hospital VP to Radiology Chair, when asked for subsidy).
- I believe we have tripled our volume since I arrived (any newly appointed Section Chief).
- One of my staff radiologists is leaving and we had an increase in interventional cases ... I need to hire two new faculty members (the same Section Chief).
- We are working harder in our section than anywhere else, and don't believe RVUs is a fair system to assess workload (any radiologist).
- With the reports you dictate it is impossible to bill! (coder).
- It takes at least 4 months to get new payer-approved radiologists; don't let them read until I tell you (billing office manager to the Chair).

Big Questions, Easy Answers

Q: We installed PACS four years ago; why are we still printing films? (Hospital COO)

A: PACS implementation does not eliminate the films in the OR, requested by referring physicians, or patient copies.
Solution: Start distributing images in CD format.

Q: Does HIPAA regulations represent a risk for my business?

A: No. Even though HIPAA has been law since 1996 and therefore being mandatory, and includes penalties for failure to comply, radiology managers concerns are limited to the enforcement of privacy and security rules to protect patients' sensitive personal information. Therefore, every radiology practice must enforce and comply with HIPAA regulations, but they do not represent a risk if information is managed appropriately.

Q: How do some imaging centers manage to serve 150 patients per day while maintaining a high level of patient satisfaction and others are able to see only 75 patients with the same level infrastructure?

A: It is all about the revenue cycle. Improvement to details regarding scheduling and registration, patient communication, staffing resources, documentation and the billing process, and reporting will ultimately produce increased productivity and profitability.

Glossary

Access: Time (days or hours) from test request to test completion. It is a key measure when deciding expansion of services.

Balanced scorecard: The balanced scorecard is a management system that enables organizations to clarify their vision and strategy and translate them into action. It provides feedback around both the internal business processes and external outcomes in order to continuously improve strategic performance and results.

Benchmarking: The process of setting goals, where these goals are chosen by comparisons with other providers, drawn from the best practices within the organization or industry. The benchmarking process identifies the best performance in the industry for a particular process or outcome, determines how that performance is achieved, and applies the lessons learned to improve performance.

Billings: Gross billed charges entered into the billing system for each CPT code.

Capitation: Method of payment for health services in which a physician or hospital is paid a fixed amount for each person served regardless of the actual number or nature of services provided.

Case-mix index (CMI): The average DRG weight for all cases paid under PPS. The CMI is a measure of the relative costliness of the patients treated in each hospital or group of hospitals (*see also* DRG).

Charge: The amount asked for a service by a health-care provider. Its contracted with the cost, which is the amount the provider incurs in furnishing the service.

Charge Lag: The number of days it takes to enter a service charge in the billing system from the date of the service.

CFTE imputed: A measure of clinical activity of an individual physician or group of physicians relative to the benchmark value for a given specialty. This is computed by dividing the actual RVUs (work or total) generated by the benchmark value selected in the report (mean, median, 75th percentile, etc).

CFTE reported: The percent of time spent in billable clinical activity, as reported by the participant. Participants must provide these data in order to calculate other measures. *Note*: if you see patients where a bill is not entered into the billing system from which data are submitted to the FPSC, you should reduce the reported CFTE by the appropriate amount.

CFTE imputed/reported: The ratio of the imputed CFTE to the reported CFTE. This ratio measures the relative productivity of providers. In other words, it tells what an individual provider or group of providers is producing compared to what is expected.

Clinical full-time equivalent (CFTE): The percent of full-time a provider spends in billable, clinical activity. Percent clinical effort cannot exceed 100%.

Cost: The value of opportunity forgone as a result of engaging resources in an activity. Note that there can be a cost without the exchange of money. $/RVU.

In considering the production process, costs may be differentiated as follows:
- *Average costs*: equivalent to the average cost per unit; i.e., the total costs divided by the total number of units of production.
- *Fixed costs*: those costs which, within a short time span, do not vary with the quantity of production; e.g., heating and lighting.
- *Incremental cost*: the extra costs associated with an expansion in activity of a given service.
- *Marginal cost*: the cost of producing one extra unit of a service.
- *Variable costs*: those costs which vary with the level of production and are proportional to quantities produced.

In considering health problems, costs may be differentiated as follows:
- *Direct costs*: those costs borne by the health-care system, community and patients' families in addressing the illness.
- *Indirect costs*: mainly productivity losses to society caused by the health problem or disease.

Cost-effectiveness analysis (CEA): An economic evaluation in which the costs and consequences of alternative interventions are expressed per unit of health outcome. CEA is used to determine technical efficiency; i.e., comparison of costs and consequences of competing interventions for a given patient group within a given budget.

CPT family: A grouping of CPT codes related to a common category of procedure (e.g., Surgery, Evaluation and management).

CPT range: A subset of codes within a CPT family that defines a particular grouping of related procedures (e.g., Surgery-Musculoskeletal).

Current procedural terminology (CPT): The coding system for physicians' services developed by the CPT Editorial Panel of the American Medical Association; basis of the HCFA Common Procedure Coding System.

Current procedural terminology code (CPT code): A systematic listing and coding of procedures and services performed by physicians. Each procedure or service is identified with a five-digit CPT code to simplify the reporting and billing of services.

Dashboard: An at-a-glance snapshot of the economic reality of the numbers inside a department. The purpose of the dashboard is to provide a tool which gives anyone the capacity to see in graphical "whole pictures" the relationships between the financial statement fragments you currently use.

Diagnosis-related groups (DRGs): A system for determining case mix, used for payment under Medicare's PPS and by some other payers. The DRG system classifies patients into groups based on the principal diagnosis, type of surgical procedure, presence or absence of significant comorbidities or complications, and other relevant criteria. DRGs are intended to categorize patients into groups that are clinically meaningful and homogeneous with respect to resource use. Medicare's PPS uses almost 500 mutually exclusive DRGs, each of which is assigned a relative weight that compares its costliness to the average for all DRGs.

Effectiveness: The net health benefits provided by a medical service or technology for typical patients in community practice settings.

Efficiency: Making the best use of available resources; i.e., getting good value for resources.

Examination volume: Number of procedures performed by time unit, e.g., CT scans per year.

Fee-for-service: The traditional method for financing health services; pays physicians and hospitals for each service they provide.

Fee schedule: A list of predetermined payment rates for medical services.

Fiscal year: A 12-month period for which an organization plans the use of its funds. FYs are referred to by the calendar year in which they end; for example, the Federal FY2006 began October 2005.

Full-time equivalent (FTE): A way to measure a worker's *productivity* and/ or involvement in a project. An FTE of 1.0 means that the person is equivalent to a full-time worker. An FTE of 0.5 may signal that the worker is only half-time, or that his projected output is only half of what one might expect.

Health maintenance organization (HMO): A managed care plan that integrates financing and delivery of a comprehensive set of health-care services to an enrolled population. HMOs may contract with, directly employ, or own participating health-care providers.

Health technology assessment: Evaluation of biomedical technology in relation to cost, efficacy, utilization, etc., and its future impact on social, ethical, and legal systems.

HIPAA (Health Insurance Portability and Accountability Act): The Administrative Simplification provisions of the Health Insurance Portability and Accountability Act of 1996 (HIPAA, title II) require the Department of Health and Human Services (HHS) to establish national standards for electronic health-care transactions and national identifiers for providers, health plans, and employers. It also addresses the security and privacy of health data. Adopting these standards will improve the efficiency and effectiveness of the nation's health-care system by encouraging the widespread use of electronic data interchange in health care.

Hospital costs: The expenses incurred by a hospital in providing care. The hospital costs attributed to a particular patient care episode include the direct costs plus an appropriate proportion of the overhead for administration, personnel, building maintenance, equipment, etc.

Hospital inpatient prospective payment system (PPS): Medicare's method of paying acute care hospitals for inpatient care. Prospective per case payment rates are set at a level intended to cover operating costs for treating a typical inpatient in a given DRG. Payments for each hospital are adjusted for differences in area wages, teaching activity, care to the poor, and other factors.

Indicator: A measure of a specific component of a health improvement strategy. An indicator can reflect an activity implemented to address a particular health issue or it might reflect outcomes from activities already implemented.

Limiting charge: The maximum amount that a nonparticipating physician is permitted to charge a Medicare beneficiary for a service: in effect, a limit on balance billing. Starting in 1993 the limiting charge has been set at 115% of the Medicare-allowed charge.

Managed care organization (MCO): Any organization that is accountable for the health of an enrolled group of people. In contrast to organizations that provide services at a discount but do not attempt to coordinate care, MCOs actually have responsibility for the health of enrollees and, as a consequence, seek improvements in both the results and cost-effectiveness of the services provided.

Management performance indicators: Indicators utilized for management of departmental activities to improve performance.

Outcome: The consequence of a medical intervention on a patient.

Outcome evaluation: Outcome evaluation is used to obtain descriptive data on a project and to document short-term results. Task-focused results are those that describe the output of the activity (e.g., the number of public inquiries received as a result of a public service announcement).

Outliers: Cases with extremely long lengths of stay (day outliers) or extraordinarily high costs (cost outliers) compared with others classified in the same diagnosis-related group.

Peer review organization (PRO): An organization that contracts with HCFA to investigate the quality of health care furnished to Medicare beneficiaries and to educate beneficiaries and providers. PROs also conduct limited review of medical records and claim to evaluate the appropriateness of care provided.

Per Diem Payments: Fixed daily payments that do not vary with the level of services used by the patient. This method generally is used to pay institutional providers, such as hospitals and nursing facilities.

Performance measure: A specific measure of how well a health plan does in providing health services to its enrolled population. Can be used as a measure of quality. Examples include mammography rate, or percentage of enrollees indicating satisfaction with care.

Performance standard: The target rate of expenditure growth set by the Volume Performance Standard system.

Practice expense relative value unit (practice expense RVU): A unit of measure used to express the amount of practice overhead costs of a service relative to other services.

Productivity: The ratio of outputs (goods and services produced) to inputs (resources used in production). Increased productivity implies that the hospital or health-care organization is either producing more output with the same resources or the same output with fewer resources.

Prospective payment: A method of paying health-care providers in which rates are established in advance. Providers are paid these rates regardless of the costs they actually incur.

Relative value unit (RVU): A non-monetary unit of measure used to express the time, complexity and cost of performing a given service relative to those of performing other procedures.

RVU/FTE ratio: A clinical productivity measure. It represents the average output of each physician, and can be used as a workload measure.

Report turnaround: Time interval between the completion of a study and the production of the final report.

Revenue: The inflow of assets that results from sales of goods and services and earnings from dividends, interest, and rent.

In $/RVU: Represents the corresponding income for each worked unit.

SCARD (Society of Chairmen in Academic Radiology Departments): Nonprofit organization dedicated to the advancement of the art and science of radiology by the promotion of medical education, research and patient care.

Spider graphs/charts: A technique or tool to combine analyses of a market's level of managed care evolution with an internal readiness review. It involves three steps: market assessment, internal analysis, and gap analysis. Components of the graph include: network formation, managed care penetration, utilization levels, reimbursement, excess inpatient capacity, geographic distribution, commercial premium, physician integration, managed care characteristics, employer and purchaser base, outcomes management, strategic alignment, organization and governance, access to markets, delivery systems, medical management, finance, performance management, and information technology.

Standard: Something set up and established by authority as a rule for the measure of quantity, weight, extent, value or quality.

Transcription time: Time measure from completion of a test to final report.

Technology adoption patterns: Organizational characteristic method of providing new technologies; e.g., innovators are considered those hospitals that develop their own technologies or that make them available to the public at an early stage.

Total relative value unit (total RVU): The value consists of three components: the physician work involved (work RVU), practice overhead costs (practice expense RVUs), and malpractice expense (malpractice RVUs). RVUs are used as the basis for reimbursement of physicians' services by Medicare and by many other third-party players.

Utilization management (UM): The process of evaluating the necessity, appropriateness, and efficiency of health-care services against established guidelines and criteria. Evaluation of the necessity, appropriateness, and efficiency of the use of health-care services, procedures, and facilities.

Utilization review (UR): The review of services delivered to evaluate appropriateness, necessity, and quality. The review can be performed on a prospective, concurrent, or retrospective basis.

Work relative value unit (work RVU): A unit of measure used to express the amount of effort (time, intensity of effort, technical skills) required of a provider in performing a given service relative to other services.

References

1. Academy for Healthcare Management (2001) Managed healthcare: an introduction, 3rd edn. Academy for Healthcare Management, Washington DC
2. AcademyHealth (2004) Glossary of terms commonly used in health care. AcademyHealth, Washington DC
3. American Association of Health Plans (1996) Capitation: questions and answers. American Association of Health Plans, Washington DC
4. American Medical Association (1993) Advocacy brief: health reform glossary. American Medical Association, Chicago, IL
5. Batstone G, Edwards M (1996) Achieving clinical effectiveness: just another initiative or a real change in working practice? J Clin Effectiveness 1(1):19–21
6. Cofer J (1985) Legislative currents: Prospective Payment Assessment Commission (ProPAC). J Am Med Rec Assoc 56(3):28
7. Dorland's Illustrated Medical Dictionary, 28th edn (1994). WB Saunders, Philadelphia
8. Drummond MF, O'Brien B, Stoddart GL, Torrance GW (1997) Methods for the economic evaluation of health care programmes, 2nd edn. Oxford University Press, Oxford
9. Kelly MP, Bacon GT, Mitchell JA (1994) Glossary of managed care terms. J Ambul Care Manage 17(1):70–76
10. Mar Queisser RL (1995) Carve-out bundled-service contracts: a new type of CBC? Northwest Physician Magazine, Spring: 26–27
11. Medicare Payment Advisory Commission (1998) Medicare Payment Policy. Report to the Congress. Medicare Payment Advisory Commission, Washington DC
12. National Library of Medicine (1994) HSTAR Fact Sheet. National Library of Medicine, Bethesda, MD
13. National Library of Medicine. Medical Subject Headings. Available at: http://www.nlm.nih.gov
14. National Library of Medicine. PubMed Tutorial Glossary. Available at: http://www.nlm.nih.gov
15. New Jersey Hospital Association (2006) Glossary of healthcare terms and abbreviations. New Jersey Hospital Association, Princeton, NJ. Available at: http://www.njha.com/publications/pubcatalog/glossary.pdf
16. Office of Technology Assessment (1993) Benefit design: clinical preventive services. Office of Technology Assessment, Washington, DC
17. Pam Pohly Associates (2006) Glossary of terms in managed health care. Pam Pohly Associates, Hays, KS. Available at: http://www.pohly.com
18. Physician Payment Review Commission (1996) Annual Report to the Congress. Physician Payment Review Commission, Washington DC
19. Pickett JP, et al (eds) (2000) The American heritage dictionary of the English language, 4th edn. Houghton Mifflin Company, Boston, MA

20. Player S (1998) Activity-based analyses lead to better decision making. Healthc Financ Manage 52(8):66–70
21. Prospective Payment Assessment Commission (ProPAC) (1996) Medicare and the American Health Care System. Report to the Congress, June 1996. Prospective Payment Assessment Commission, Washington, DC
22. Rhea JC, Ott JS, Shafritz JM (1988) The facts on file dictionary of health care management. Facts on File Publications, New York, NY
23. Rossi PH, Freeman HE (1993) Evaluation: a systematic approach. Sage Publications, Newbury Park
24. Scott DL (2003) Wall Street words: an A to Z guide to investment terms for today's investor. Houghton Mifflin Company, Boston, MA
25. Timmreck TC (1997) Health services cyclopedic dictionary: a compendium of health-care and public health terminology. Jones and Bartlett, Sudbury, MA
26. Tufts Managed Care Institute (1996) Managed care at a glance: common terms, 6. Tufts Managed Care Institute, Boston, MA
27. Turnock J (2001) Public health, what it is and how it works. Aspen, Gaithersburg, MD
28. US Congressional Budget Office (1988) Including capital expenses in the prospective payment system. Congress of the United States, Washington DC
29. Washington State Department of Health (1994) Public Health Improvement Plan: a progress report. Olympia, WA
30. World Bank (2001) Health systems development. Health Economics. World Bank, Washington DC
31. Zarnke KB, Levine MA, O'Brien BJ (1997) Cost-benefit analyses in the health-care literature: don't judge a study by its label. J Clin Epidemiol 50(7):813–822
32. http://www.financialscoreboard.com/dashboard.html
33. http://www.cms.hhs.gov/HIPAAGenInfo

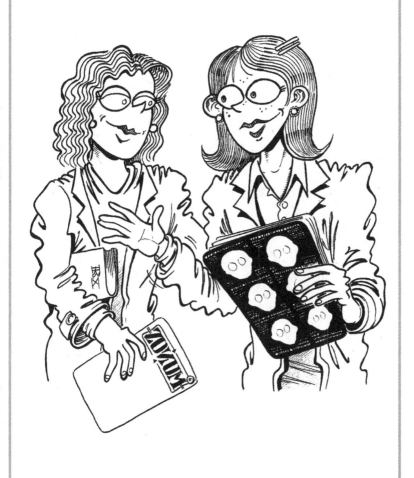

Unit XVII   Radiological Conversation Guide

With this guide we intend to provide radiologists with useful sentences, expressions, abbreviations, and acronyms frequently used in different radiological settings. You, as radiology resident, fellow or attending, must create your own conversation guide with sentences frequently used at your institution. Medical and radiological jargon is so institution-specific that unless you belong to a particular institution you will not understand some terms and expressions used in that institution.

Medical language is complex and colorful. To address all radiological terms and expressions is beyond the scope of this, and probably any, work. Instead, this compilation focuses on terms and expressions not specifically described in textbooks which have, over time, become part of the medical language. Many of these terms are well known to a person who has trained in an English-speaking environment but may not be familiar to others. Some of the terms and expressions are encountered within radiology, while others are more often used by non-radiologists but make their way into our interactions with our colleagues and as part of medical histories. The unit is divided into four sections:

1. Conversational abbreviations
2. Conversational acronyms
3. Made-up words/definitions/expressions
4. Conversational scenarios

Let there be no misunderstanding: those terms marked with a *double asterisk*, although used covertly, are not appropriate for use openly in any circumstances; other terms with no asterisk may not be appropriate in some circumstances. If in doubt about a slang term, do not use it.

Conversational Abbreviations

Appy	Appendectomy
Art line	Arterial line
Bili	Bilirubin
Bx	Biopsy
Cathed	Catheterized

Crit	Hematocrit
DC	Discontinue (or) discharge
Di-di pregnancy	Dichorionic-diamniotic twin gestation
Ex lap	Exploratory laparotomy
Lap chole	Laparoscopic cholecystectomy
Lytes	Electrolytes
Preemie	Premature infant
Scope	To undergo endoscopy
Scope from above	EGD
Scope from below	Colonoscopy
Tics	Diverticulae

Conversational Acronyms

ALC**	"a la casa" – to send the patient home
CABG (pronounced cabbage)	Coronary artery bypass graft
CCU	Coronary care unit
CP	chest pain
DNR	Do not resuscitate
DVT	Deep venous thrombus
EGD	Esophagogastroduodenoscopy
ERCP	Endoscopic retrograde cholangiopancreatography
KUB	"Kidney ureters bladder" – abdominal radiograph
GNR	Gram-negative rod bacteria
LAD	Lymphadenopathy
LFTs	Liver function tests
MI	Myocardial infarction
MRSA	Methicillin-resistant *Staphylococcus aureus*
NAD	No acute distress
NICU	Neurosurgical intensive care unit, or Neonatal intensive care unit, depending on context
POD	Postoperative day (followed by number)
ROMI	"Rule out myocardial infarction" – evaluation of a patient suspected of suffering from a heart attack; can be used as a verb
SICU (pronounced "sick-U")	Surgical intensive care unit
STEMI	ST wave elevated myocardial infarction
TAH/BSO	Total abdominal hysterectomy/bilateral salpingoophorectomy
UA	Urinalysis, or uric acid, depending on context
USOH	Usual state of health; for example: "Pt was in USOH until 2 weeks ago when ..."

V-fib	Ventricular fibrillation
WADAO**	"Weak and dizzy all over"

Made-Up Words/Definitions/Expressions

Albatross**	Chronically ill patient who will remain with a doctor until one of them expires
Ax or blade or sturgeon**	Surgeon
Aunt Minnie lesion	Once seen, never forgotten, much like certain aunts at the family wedding. Processes with distinct and unique imaging features that allow diagnosis without differential
Babygram	Whole body radiograph of a newborn
Big C**	Cancer
Boogie or goober**	Tumor
Bordeaux**	Urine with blood in it
Bounceback	Patient who keeps returning to the hospital, a short time after discharge
Box**	To die
Bronk	To undergo bronchoscopy
Buff up	To ready a patient for release
Bug juice	Antibiotics
Champagne tap	Reference to the bottle of sparkling wine a junior resident should receive from his consultant after achieving a bloodless lumbar puncture
Code brown	Fecal incontinence emergency
Code yellow	Urinary incontinence emergency
Dermaholiday**	Nickname for dermatology department used by staff in busier departments
Doc-in-the-box**	Small urgent care medical facility, usually in a shopping center, where one can go for treatment without an appointment
Donorcycle**	Motorbike: frequent cause of organ donation
Dr. Feelgood**	A doctor who is indiscriminate about prescribing drugs, particularly narcotics
Fake-oma or fakeout	Imaging finding that mimics pathology or abnormality but is in fact normal
Fascinoma	A "fascinating" tumor or pathological process, notable for it's rarity or unusual presentation
Frequent flier	Patient, usually of the ER, who frequently returns for care and is known by many employees of the service

Gomergram**	Ordering all available tests because the person is unable to explain what is wrong with them or because symptoms are too vague to form a reasonable differential. Also see "shotgun approach"
Incidentaloma	Imaging or lab finding made while searching or working-up a patient for an unrelated process
O sign**	Comatose patient with mouth open wide
Q sign**	An O sign with the patient's tongue hanging out – a worse prognosis
Retrospectoscope	Viewing a past case with the benefit of hindsight
Scut	A noun or a verb, referring to work that medical students or lower-level residents have to do which does not offer any learning opportunity, but needs to get done
Scut monkey**	Person who performs more than his/her fair share of scut
Shotgun approach (Shotgunning)	Ordering of a vast array of tests or imaging studies in the hope that something will give an idea of what is wrong with the patient
Shrink**	Psychiatrist
St. Elsewhere**	Medical academia's term for any non-teaching hospital
Supratentorial**	Literally means above the falx tentorium/cerebellum, but is often used to imply a psychosomatic or imagined process
Train wreck**	A patient with many serious medical problems
Turf**	To move a patient to a different service, as in "Turf that woman in the ER to obstetrics". Also, administrative/political conflict over division of certain procedures by department
Vitamin H	Haldol
Wall	Intern or resident adept at not admitting patients to his or her service
Zebra	An unusually strange or unexpected disease (from the saying "When you hear hoofbeats, the smart money is on horses, not zebras")

Conversational Scenarios

Radiologist preparing to perform an ultrasound on two-year-old Eric:

- *Radiologist*: "Good morning Mr. and Mrs. Brown (patient's parents). I am the radiologist, Dr. Miller. I'd like to talk to you about the examination I am about to perform on Eric (patient). Based on Eric's symptoms of projectile vomiting, it is believed that he may have a hypertrophic pyloric stenosis. This is a condition that can be established by ultrasound. We can discuss the condition later in more detail but for now I would like to focus on the ultrasound examination. The ultrasound examination is a non-invasive technique used to image structures by using sound waves. Sometimes, pressure from the ultrasound probe may cause discomfort, but the sound waves themselves cause no pain or damage to the tissue. Do you have any questions? ..."

Patient, Mrs. Belmont, has questions regarding oral and intravenous contrast:

- *Technologist*: "Dr. Miller (radiologist), Mrs. Belmont (patient) is refusing to drink the oral contrast because it tastes badly and she has questions about potential complications from the intravenous contrast. She wishes to speak to the radiologist."
- *Radiologist, speaking to patient*: "Good morning Mrs. Belmont. I am the radiologist, Dr. Miller. It's a pleasure to meet you. Our technologist has told me of your concern regarding both the oral and intravenous contrast. I would like to address your questions. Let me begin by saying that the choice to accept or refuse oral and intravenous contrast is entirely yours to make. However, I would like to convey to you the importance of contrast. It is a tool that enables us to obtain more information from the CT and makes the examination more useful. Allergic reactions can be mild to severe, but in your case, you have no history of allergic reaction (had past contrast-enhanced CT without adverse reaction) and no renal insufficiency so the risk of damage to your kidneys is minimal. Some patients describe a warm sensation as the contrast is administered, but that is normal and expected. Ultimately, the choice is yours but in this case, the benefits of using contrast are greater than the risks."

Talking to referral physician:

- *Radiologist*: "Good morning Dr. Clark. I just reviewed your patient's, Mrs. Tall's, CT and wanted to discuss the findings with you ..."
- *Radiologist*: " Good morning Dr. Clark. I am reviewing Mrs. Tall's abdominal CT and am hoping to obtain more information on her presentation and past surgical history ..."
- *Radiologist*: "Dr. Clark, Thank you for contacting me regarding Mrs. Tall's CT. I received the prior studies from Memorial Hospital and have been able to compare them with our most recent studies. There has been no significant interval change in the appearance of the 2 cm liver lesion in segment VI. I suspect it may be a hemangioma. If that is the area of concern, the next study of choice would be a multiphase CT or MR with dynamic sequences ..."

Radiologist, speaking to mammography technologist:

- "Thelma (technologist), I just reviewed Mrs. Smith's MLO and CC views. There is an asymmetric density in the upper outer quadrant, seen on the MLO view only. I'd like to get a spot compression in the ML projection."

Talking to CT/MR technician:

- *Radiologist*: "Jim (technologist), can you reconstruct the upper abdomen from the liver dome to the celiac trunk in 1×5's? I would like the images reformatted in the sagittal and coronal plane as well."

Talking to patient:

- *Mr. Jones*: "Doctor, will this hurt?"
- *Dr. Smith*: "We will use two different types of medication to make the procedure as comfortable as possible. The first type of medication is part of what is called intravenous conscious sedation. The medication will be given to you through your IV line. One of the medications is for pain and the other will make you a little sleepy. In addition to the medication through your IV, we will also be injecting a local anesthetic medication at the site of the procedure. That medication is similar to what you receive at the dentist. It will make the skin numb. It may hurt briefly at the very beginning but should not hurt once the medication starts working which will take about one minute. As you will be awake, you can let us know if you feel pain during the procedure and more medication will be given to you."

Radiologist preparing for procedure:

- *Technologist*: "Dr. Smith, Mr. Jones is on the table. Should I start prepping?" (Prepping includes application of Betadine and placement of sterile drapes.)
- *Dr. Smith*: "Yes, please start prepping. I'll go scrub." (Scrubbing is the process of meticulously cleaning one's hands with a scrub sponge.)
- *Technologist*: "I'll have your gown ready for you. What size gloves do you take?"
- *Dr. Smith*: "I take 8s. Thanks."

Talking to a patient about recovery and discharge:

- *Dr. Smith*: "Mr. Jones, everything went well during the procedure and the results of the biopsy will be available in a few days. How are you feeling?"
- *Mr. Jones*: "I am a little sleepy but fine otherwise."
- *Dr. Smith*: "Good. As part of our standard protocol we would like to keep you in recovery for 6 hours. Your wife is in the waiting area and

will be joining you shortly. Remember that you should not drive, operate machinery or take part in any activity that is strenuous or requires physical or mental effort for the rest of the day. The medication you have received will keep you drowsy for a few hours. As part of your discharge packet, there is a list of signs and symptoms that you should be aware of. I'll go over the list with you. Here is my phone number. Do not hesitate to contact me if you have any questions or concerns."

Obtaining informed consent:

- *Dr. Smith*: "Good morning Mr. Jones, I am Dr. Smith. I would like to discuss the procedure planned for this morning. Let me begin by briefly going over your past medical history and current concerns ... (Going over a patient's medical history establishes a rapport and link that radiologists often don't have with patients. It places the procedure in the proper context and shows that the interventional radiologist's range extends beyond just doing a procedure.) ... Please feel free to correct any information I have or to add any information you feel is relevant.
  Let me then give you an overview of the procedure. You will not be completely asleep for the procedure, so I will talk to you as we proceed [*Describe procedure*]. Do you have any questions thus far? (You can ask the patient to re-explain the procedure to you in their own words to ensure that they understand. We often use technical terms without recognizing that most people are not familiar with those terms.)
  As with any procedure, there are certain risks and alternatives [*List or describe risks and alternatives of the procedure*]. Some of the risks I described may seem worrisome but it's important to keep them in the proper context. We would not offer the procedure unless we thought that the benefits of the procedure outweigh the risks.
  Do you have any questions?"

Radiologist asking about an ICU patient undergoing an abdominal US scan:

- *Radiologist*: "Is patient intubated? Can patient be repositioned in both right and left lateral decubitus positions?"
- *Nurse*: "Yes, patient is intubated but can be turned about 30 degrees. I will get some extra help to move the patient. Transport is on the way."

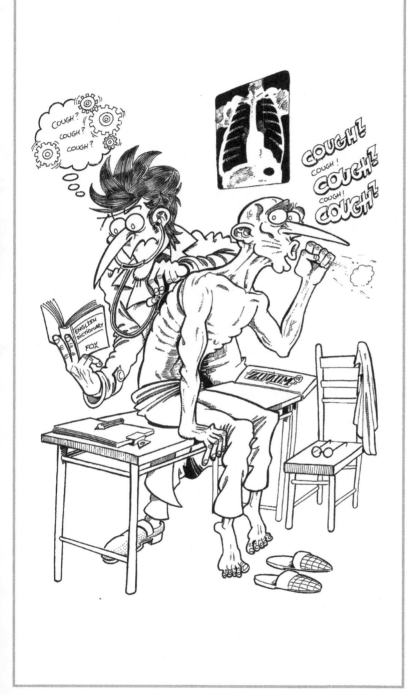

Unit XVIII Basic Communication Skills in Medicine

In the following pages we show several key sentences which can help you when interviewing a patient. In Table 1 we provide a list of common phrases that patients use to describe their symptoms, and the meaning of these phrases.

Greeting and Introducing Yourself

- Good afternoon, Mr. Hudson. I'm Dr. Smith. How may I help you?
- Good morning, Mr. Lee. Come and sit down. I'm Dr. Walker.
- Good afternoon, Mrs. Belafonte. Take a seat, please.
- Good afternoon, Mrs. Belafonte. I'm Dr. Smith. The technician told me you wanted to talk to the radiologist.

Invitation to Describe Symptoms

- Well now, what seems to be the problem?
- What brought you in today?
- Well, how can I help you?
- Would you please tell me how I can help you?
- Have you been having trouble with your blood pressure lately?
- Where does your knee hurt?
- Does lying down help the pain?
- Does standing up make it worse?
- What's the pain like?
- What kind of pain is it?
- Can you describe your pain?
- Does anything make it worse?
- Is there anything else you feel at the same time?
- Is there anything that makes it better?
- How long does the pain last?
- Have you taken anything for it?
- Your GP (general practitioner) says you've been having trouble with your right shoulder. Tell me about it.

Table 1. Common phrases used by patients, and their meaning

When a patient says ...	The doctor understands ...
I can't breath or I'm stuffed up or my chest is tight	Dyspnea
Everything is spinning	Vertigo
It itches or I'm itching	Pruritus
It stings when I pee	Dysuria
I can't eat or I've lost my appetite	Anorexia
I don't feel like doing anything	Asthenia
Headache	Cephalgia
My nose is dripping	Rhinorrhea
I've vaginal dripping	Leukorrhea
I'm having my period	Menstruation
My hair is falling out	Alopecia
I can't remember a thing	Amnesia
My skin looks yellow	Jaundice
I can't move (a limb)	Paralysis
I can't see anything	Blindness
Bad breath	Halitosis
I've a cavity	Caries
It hurts when I swallow	Odynophagia
I can't swallow	Dysphagia
I spit out phlegm (when I cough)	Sputum
Cough up blood	Hemoptysis
My stomach is burning	Epigastralgia
I wheeze	Wheeze
I've a prickly sensation	Paresthesia
I've a burning sensation	Pyrosis
I feel like I'm going to throw up	Nausea
I'm always running to the bathroom	Polyuria
I always feel like I have to pee	Tenesmus
I'm always thirsty or I'm always dry	Polydipsia
I've a rash	Erythema
My ... is swollen	Edema
My skin looks blue	Cyanosis
My chest feels constricted	Thoracic pain
My mouth is always watering	Sialorrhea
I can't breathe when I lie down	Orthopnea
My stool is black	Melena
My stool is white	Acholia
My urine is dark	Choluria
I can't sleep	Insomnia
I can't go to the bathroom	Anuria
Bruise	Hematoma
Toothache	Odontalgia

- My colleague, Dr. Sanders, says your left knee has been aching lately. Is that correct?
- Have you had any pain in your ...?
- Have you ever coughed up blood?
- Have you had any shortness of breath?
- Any pain in your muscles?
- Have you lost any weight?
- Do you suffer from double vision?

Instructions for Undressing

- Would you slip off your top things, please?
- Slip off your coat, please?
- Would you mind taking off all your clothes except your underwear? (men)
- Please would you take off all your clothes except your underwear and bra? (women)
- You should take off your underwear too.
- Lie on the couch and cover yourself with the blanket.
- Lie on the stretcher with your shoes and socks off, please.
- Roll your sleeve up, please, I'm going to examine your elbow.

Instructions for Position on Couch

- Make yourself comfortable on the couch and lie on your back (supine position).
- Lie down, please (supine position).
- Roll over onto your tummy (from supine to prone position).
- Lie on your tummy, please (prone position).
- Please turn over and lie on your back again.
- Bend your left knee.
- Straighten your leg again.
- Roll over onto your right side.
- Keep the knee straight.
- Sit with your legs dangling over the edge of the couch.
- Lie down with your legs stretched out in front of you.
- Sit up and bend you knees.
- Lean forward.
- Get off the stretcher ("Get off" is sometimes perceived as too informal and impolite).
- Please come off the couch.
- Please sit up.
- Get off the couch and stand up ("Get off" is sometimes perceived as too informal and impolite).

- Stand up from the couch.
- Stand up, please.
- Lie on your back with your knees bent and your legs wide apart.
- Lie on your tummy and relax.
- Let yourself go loose.

Instructions to Get Dressed

- You can get dressed now. Take your time, we are not in a hurry.
- Please get dressed. Take your time, we are not in a hurry.

No Treatment

- There is nothing wrong with you (It may be a quirk of the US health-care system, but we are encouraged to validate a patient's complaints. Hence, even if nothing objective is identified, the patient's symptoms are still acknowledged. For example, I might say "I understand that you have back pain. The MRI does not show any abnormality or anything that requires treatment. Our next step will be to ...")
- This will clear up on its own.
- This illness is self-limited and will resolve on its own.
- There doesn't seem to be anything wrong with your shoulder.

Questions and Commands

- To begin the interview:
  - Well now, how can I help you?
  - What's brought you in today?
  - What can I do for you?
  - What seems to be the problem?
  - Well, Mr. Goyen, what's the trouble?
  - Your doctor says you've been having trouble with your knees. Tell me about it.
  - How long has/have it/they been bothering you?
  - How long have you had it/them?
  - How long have you been ill?
  - Did it start all of a sudden?
  - How many days have you been indisposed?
  - What do you think the reason is?
  - Do you think there is any explanation?

- General questions/commands:
  - How many times?
  - How much?
  - How often?
  - How old are you?
  - Have you had bleeding?
  - Have you had fever?
  - Have you had any nose bleeding?
  - Have you lost weight lately?
  - Open your mouth, please.
  - Please remove your clothing.
  - Raise your arm.
  - Raise it more.
  - Say it once again.
  - Stick out your tongue.
  - Swallow please.
  - Take a deep breath.
  - Breathe normally.
  - Grasp my hand.
  - Try again.
  - Bear down as if for a bowel movement (Valsalva's maneuver).
  - Please lie on your tummy (prone position).
  - Please turn over and lie on your back.
  - Roll over onto your right/left side.
  - Bend your knees.
  - Keep your right knee bent.
  - Lean forward.
  - Walk across the room.
  - You can get dressed now. There's no hurry. Take your time.

Common Symptom Areas

Pain

- Questions:
  - Which part of your (head, arm, face, chest, ...) is affected?
  - Where does it hurt?
  - Where is it sore?
  - Can you describe the pain?
  - What is the pain like?
  - Is your pain severe?
  - What kind of pain are you experiencing?
  - Is there anything that makes it better?
  - Does anything make it worse?
  - Does anything relieve the pain?

- What effect does food have?
- Does lying down help the pain?
• Describing the characteristics of pain:
    - A dull sort of pain.
    - A feeling of pressure.
    - Very sore, like a knife.
    - A burning pain.
    - A gnawing kind of pain.
    - A sharp, stabbing pain.
    - Raw.
    - The pain's gone.
    - A sharp pain.
    - I ache all over.
    - I'm in a lot of pain.
    - I've got a very sore arm.

Fever

- I think I have a temperature.
- I think I'm running a fever.
- High fever.
- High temperature.
- When do you have the highest temperature?
- Do you shiver?
- Do you have chills?
- Were you cold last night?
- When does your temperature come down?

Sickness

- I feel queasy.
- I feel sick.
- I think I'm going to vomit.
- I think I'm going to throw everything up.
- My head is (swimming) spinning.
- I feel dizzy.
- He's feeling giddy.
- She's feeling faint.

Weakness

- I feel weak.
- I'm tired.

- I'm not in the mood for ...
- Are you hungry?
- I've lost weight.
- Do you still feel very weak?

Sleep

- Do you feel sleepy?
- Do you sleep deeply?
- I wake up too early.
- Do you snore?

Vision

- I can't see properly.
- Everything is fuzzy.
- Everything is blurred.
- I can't see with my left/right eye.
- My eye is itchy.
- My eye is stinging/burning.
- What have you done to your eye?
- What's happened to your eye?

Others

- Have you had a cough?
- Do you pass any blood?
- Do you have a discharge?
- My foot has gone to sleep.
- The patient went into a coma.

Key Words About Symptoms and Signs

General Symptoms

- Malaise
- Anorexia (no appetite)
- Weakness
- Vomiting (throw up)
- Myalgia
- Muscle pain

- Sweats
- Weight loss
- Weight gain
- Drowsiness
- Night sweats
- Insomnia
- Chills
- Numbness
- Tingling
- Fever
- Constipation
- Regular movements
- Diarrhea

Skin

- Rash
- Lump
- Pruritus
- Itch
- Scar
- Bruising
- Spots
- Blackhead
- Moles
- Swelling
- Puffiness
- Tingle

Respiratory System

- Cough
- Productive cough
- Unproductive cough
- Hemoptysis
- Cough up blood
- Cough up phlegm or spit
- Coryza
- Runny nose
- Sputum
- Sore throat
- Pleuritic pain
- Dyspnea
- Breathlessness

- Out of puff
- Chest pain
- Orthopnea
- Breathless on lying down

Cardiovascular System

- Chest pain
- Pain behind the breast bone
- Intermittent claudication
- Cramps
- Palpitations
- Angina
- Tachycardia
- Cyanosis

Gastrointestinal System

- Abdominal pain
- Nausea
- Vomitus
- Vomit
- Diarrhea
- Constipation
- Flatulence
- A coated tongue

Genitourinary System

- Polyuria
- Dysuria
- Pollakiuria
- Tenesmus
- Leukorrhea
- Menorrhagia
- Dysmenorrhea
- Impotence
- Frigidity
- Menstrual cramps

Nervous System

- Tremor
- Rigidity
- Seizure
- Paralysis
- Palsy
- Paresthesia
- Reflex
- Ataxia
- Incontinence
- Jumbled speech
- Knee jerk

Patient Examination

Initial Examination

- Level of consciousness:
  - Altered level of consciousness
  - GCS (Glasgow coma scale)
  - Loss of consciousness
  - Alert and oriented

- Circulation:
  - Heart tones/sounds
  - Clear
  - Distant
  - Regular/Irregular
  - Muffled
  - Pulse

- Breathing:
  - Rhythm
  - Depth
  - Adequate
  - Shallow
  - Deep
  - Quality
  - Easy
  - Labored
  - Stridor
  - Painful
  - Shortness of breath

Systematic Examination

- Respiratory system:
  - Breathing
  - Regular
  - Easy
  - Shallow
  - Deep
  - Non-productive cough
  - Productive cough
  - Chest auscultation
  - Mucus and pink nail beds
  - Telltale stains

- Cardiovascular system:
  - No abnormalities in heart rate or rhythm
  - Peripheral pulses
  - Normal color and temperature of skin
  - No ankle edema

- Gastrointestinal system:
  - Abdomen soft, non-tender
  - No nausea or vomiting
  - No abnormalities in stool patterns or characteristics
  - No change in dietary patterns
  - Bowel sounds present

- Genitourinary system:
  - No abnormalities in voiding patterns
  - No abnormalities in color or characteristics of urine
  - No vaginal or penile drainage

- Nervous system:
  - Finger to finger
  - Finger to nose

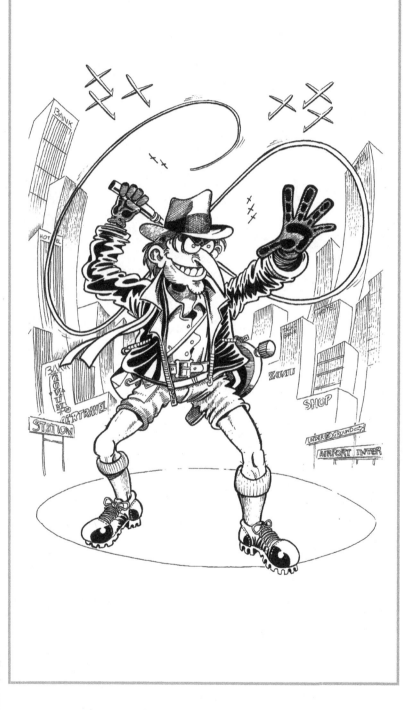

Unit XIX Conversation Survival Guide

Introduction

Fluency gives self-confidence and its lack undermines you.

The intention of this unit is not to replace conversation guides; on the contrary, we encourage you, according to your level, to use them.

Without including translations, it would have been foolish to write a conversation guide. Why, then, have we written this unit? The aim of the unit is to provide a "survival guide", a basic tool, to be reviewed by upper-intermediate speakers who are actually perfectly able to understand all the usual exchanges, but can have some difficulty in finding natural ways to express themselves in certain unusual scenarios. For instance, we are strolling with a colleague who wants us to accompany him to a jeweler's to buy a bracelet for his wife. Bear in mind that, even in your own language, fluency is virtually impossible in all situations. I have only been upset and disappointed (in English) three times. At a laundry, at an airport, and, on a third occasion, at a restaurant. I considered myself relatively fluent in English by that time but, under pressure, thoughts come to mind much faster than words and your level of fluency can be overwhelmed as a consequence of the adrenaline levels in your blood. Accept this piece of advice: unless you are bilingual you cannot afford to get into arguments in a language other than your own.

Many upper-intermediate speakers do not take a conversation guide when traveling abroad. They think their level is well above those who need a guide to construct basic sentences and are ashamed of being seen reading one (I myself went through this stage). I was (and they are) utterly wrong in not taking a guide because, for upper-intermediate speakers, a conversation guide has different and very important uses (as my level increased, I realized that my use of these guides changed; I did not need to read the translations, except for a few words, and I just looked for natural ways of saying things).

In my opinion, even for those who are bilingual, conversation guides are extremely helpful whenever you are in an unfamiliar environment such as, for example, a florist. How many names of flowers do you know in your own language? Probably fewer than a dozen. Think that every conversation scenario has its own jargon and a conversation guide can give you the hints that an upper-intermediate speaker may need to be actually fluent in many situations. So, do not be ashamed of carrying and reading a guide, even in public; they are the shortest way to fluency in those unfamiliar scenarios that sporadically test our English level and, what is more important, our self-confidence in English.

Whenever you have to go out to dinner, for example, review the key words and usual sentences of your conversation guide. It will not take more than ten minutes, and your dinner will taste even better since you have ordered it with unbelievable fluency and precision. What is just a recommendable task for upper-intermediate speakers is absolutely mandatory for lower-intermediate speakers who, before leaving the hotel, should review, and rehearse the sentences they will need to ask for whatever they want to eat or, at least, to avoid ordering what they never would eat in their own country. Looking at the faces of your colleagues once the first course is served you will realize who is eating what he wanted and who, on the contrary, does not know what he ordered and, what is worse, what he is actually eating.

Let us think for a moment about this incident that happened to me when I was at UCSF Medical Center. I was invited to have lunch at a diner near the hospital, and when I asked for still mineral water, the somewhat surprised waiter answered that they did not have still mineral water but sparkling because no customer had ever asked for such a "delicacy" and offered me plain water instead. (If you do not understand this story, the important words to look up in the dictionary are diner, with one "n", still, sparkling, and plain.)

Would you be fluent without the help of a guide in a car breakdown? I did have a leak in the gas tank on a trip with my wife and mother-in-law from Boston to Niagara Falls and Toronto. I still remember the face of the mechanic in Toronto when asking me if we were staying in downtown Toronto. I answered that we were on our way back to … Boston. I can tell you that my worn guide was vital, without it I would not have been able to explain what the problem was. This was the last time I had to take the guide from a hidden pocket in my suitcase. Since then I have kept my guide with me, even at … the beach, because unexpected situations may arise at any time by definition. Think of possibly embarrassing, although not infrequent, situations and … do not forget your guide on your next trip abroad (the inside pocket of your jacket is a suitable place for those who still have not overcome the stage of "guide-ashamedness").

Those who have reached a certain level are aware of the many embarrassing situations they have had to overcome in the past to become fluent in a majority of circumstances.

Greetings

- Hi.
- Hello.
- Good morning.
- Good afternoon.
- Good evening.
- Good night.
- How are you? (Very) Well, thank you.
- How are you getting on? All right, thank you.
- I am glad to see you.
- Nice to see you (again).
- How do you feel today?
- How is your family?
- Good bye.
- Bye bye.
- See you later.
- See you soon.
- See you tomorrow.
- Give my regards to everybody.
- Give my love to your children.

Presentations

- This is Mr./Mrs. ...
- These are Mister and Missis ...
- My name is ...
- What is your name? My name is ...
- Pleased/Nice to meet you.
- Let me introduce you to ...
- I'd like to introduce you to ...
- Have you already met Mr. ...? Yes, I have.

Personal Data

- What is your name? My name is ...
- What is your surname/family name? My surname/family name is ...
- Where are you from? I am from ...
- Where do you live? I live in ...
- What is your address? My address is ...
- What is your email address? My email address is ...

- What is your phone number? My phone number is ...
- What is your mobile phone/cellular number? My mobile phone/cellular number is ...
- How old are you? I am ...
- Where were you born? I was born in ...
- What do you do? I am a radiologist.
- What do you do? I do MRI/US/CT/chest ...

Courtesy Sentences

- Thank you very much. You are welcome (don't mention it).
- Would you please ...? Sure, it is a pleasure.
- Excuse me.
- Pardon.
- Sorry.
- Cheers!
- Congratulations!
- Good luck!
- It doesn't matter!
- May I help you?
- Here you are?
- You are very kind. It is very kind of you.
- Don't worry, that's not what I wanted.
- Sorry to bother/trouble you.
- Don't worry!
- What can I do for you?
- How can I help you?
- Would you like something to drink?
- Would you like a cigarette?
- I would like ...
- I beg your pardon.
- Have a nice day.

Speaking in a Foreign Language

- Do you speak English/Spanish/French ...? I do not speak English/Only a bit/Not a word.
- Do you understand me? Yes, I do. No, I don't.
- Sorry, I do not understand you.
- Could you speak slowly, please?
- How do you write it?
- Could you write it down?

- How do you spell it?
- How do you pronounce it?
- Sorry, what did you say?
- Sorry, my English is not very good.
- Sorry, I didn't get that.
- Could you please repeat that?
- I can't hear you.

At the Restaurant

"The same for me" is one of the most common sentences heard at tables around the world. The non-fluent English speaker links his/her gastronomic fate to a reportedly more fluent one in order to avoid uncomfortable counter-questions such as "How would you like your meat, sir?"

A simple look at a guide a few minutes before the dinner will provide you with enough vocabulary to ask for whatever you want.

Do not let your lack of fluency spoil a good opportunity to taste delicious dishes or wines.

Preliminary Exchanges

- Hello, have you got a table for three people?
- Hi, may I book a table for a party of seven at 6 o'clock?
- What time are you coming, sir?
- Where can we sit?
- Is this chair free?
- Is this table taken?
- Waiter/waitress, I would like to order.
- Could I see the menu?
- Could you bring the menu?
- Can I have the wine list?
- Could you give us a table next to the window?
- Could you give me a table on the mezzanine?
- Could you give us a table near the stage?

Ordering

- We'd like to order now.
- Could you bring us some bread, please?
- We'd like to have something to drink.
- Here you are.
- Could you recommend a local wine?

- Could you recommend one of your specialties?
- Could you suggest something special?
- What are the ingredients of this dish?
- I'll have a steamed lobster, please.
- How would you like your meat, sir?
- Rare/medium-rare/medium/well-done.
- Somewhere between rare and medium rare will be OK.
- Is the halibut fresh?
- What is there for dessert?
- Anything else, sir?
- No, we are fine, thank you.
- The same for me.
- Enjoy your meal, sir.
- How was everything, sir?
- The meal was excellent.
- The sirloin was delicious.
- Excuse me, I have spilt something on my tie. Could you help me?

Complaining

- The dish is cold. Would you please heat it up?
- The meat is underdone. Would you cook it a little more, please?
- Excuse me. This is not what I asked for.
- Could you change this for me?
- The fish is not fresh. I want to see the manager.
- I asked for a sirloin.
- The meal wasn't very good.
- The meat smells off.
- Could you bring the complaints book?
- This wine is off, I think ...
- Waiter, this fork is dirty.

The Check (The Bill)

- The check, please.
- Would you bring us the check, please?
- All together, please.
- We are paying separately.
- I am afraid there is a mistake, we didn't have this.
- This is for you.
- Keep the change.

City Transportation

- I want to go to the Metropolitan museum.
- Which bus/tram/underground line must I take for the Metropolitan?
- Which bus/tram/underground line can I take to get to the Metropolitan?
- Where does the number ... bus stop?
- Does this bus go to ...?
- How much is a single ticket?
- Three tickets, please.
- Where must I get off for ...?
- Is this seat occupied/vacant?
- Where can I get a taxi?
- How much is the fare for ...?
- Take me to ... Street.
- Do you know where the ... is?

Shopping

Asking About Store Hours

- When are you open?
- How late are you open today?
- Are you open on Saturday?

Preliminary Exchanges

- Hello sir (madam), may I help you?
- Can I help you find something?
- Thank you, I am just looking.
- I just can't make up my mind.
- Can I help you with something?
- If I can help you, just let me know.
- Are you looking for something in particular?
- I am looking for something for my wife.
- I am looking for something for my husband.
- I am looking for something for my children.
- It is a gift.
- Hi, do you sell ...?
- I am looking for a ... Can you help me?
- Would you tell me where the music department is?
- Which floor is the leather goods department on? On the ground floor (on the mezzanine, on the second floor ...)

- Please would you show me ...?
- What kind do you want?
- Where can I find the mirror? There is a mirror over there.
- The changing rooms are over there.
- Only four items are allowed in the dressing room at a time.
- Is there a public rest room here?
- Have you decided?
- Have you made up your mind?

Buying Clothes/Shoes

- Please, can you show me some natural silk ties?
- I want to buy a long-sleeved shirt.
- I want the pair of high-heeled shoes I have seen in the window.
- Would you please show me the pair in the window?
- What material is it?
- What material is it made of? Cotton, leather, linen, wool, velvet, silk, nylon, acrylic fiber.
- What size, please?
- What size do you need?
- Is this my size?
- Do you think this is my size?
- Where is the fitting room?
- Does it fit you?
- I think it fits well although the collar is a little tight.
- No, it doesn't fit me.
- May I try a larger size?
- I'll try a smaller size. Would you mind bringing it to me?
- I'll take this one.
- How much is it?
- This is too expensive.
- Oh, this is a bargain!
- I like it.
- May I try this on?
- In which color? Navy blue, please.
- Do you have anything to go with this?
- I need a belt/a pair of socks/pair of jeans/pair of gloves ...
- I need a size 38.
- I don't know my size. Can you measure me?
- Would you measure my waist, please?
- Do you have a shirt to match this?
- Do you have this in blue/in wool/in a larger size/in a smaller size?
- Do you have something a bit less expensive?
- I'd like to try this on. Where is the fitting room?
- How would you like to pay for this? Cash/credit

- We don't have that in your size/color.
- We are out of that item.
- It's too tight/loose
- It's too expensive/cheap
- I don't like the color.
- Is it in the sale?
- Can I have this gift wrapped?

At the Shoe Shop

- A pair of shoes, boots, sandals, slippers ..., shoelace, sole, heel, leather, suede, rubber, shoehorn.
- What kind of shoes do you want?
- I want a pair of rubber-soled shoes/high-heeled shoes/leather shoes/ suede slippers/boots.
- I want a pair of lace-up/slip-on shoes good for the rain/for walking.
- What is your size, please?
- They are a little tight/too large/too small.
- Would you please show me the pair in the window?
- Can I try a smaller/larger size, please?
- This one fits well.
- I would like some polish cream.
- I need some new laces
- I need a shoe-horn.

At the Post Office

- I need some (first class) stamps, please.
- First class, please.
- Air mail, please.
- I would like this to go express mail.
- I would like this recorded/special delivery.
- I need to send this second-day mail (US).
- Second-class for this, please (UK).
- I need to send this parcel post.
- I need to send this by certified mail.
- I need to send this by registered mail.
- Return receipt requested, please.
- How much postage do I need for this?
- How much postage do I need to send this air mail?
- Do you have any envelopes?
- How long will it take to get there? It should arrive on Monday.
- The forms are over there. Please fill out (UK fill in) a form and bring it back to me.

Going to the Theater (*UK* Theatre)

- Sorry, we are sold out tonight.
- Sorry, these tickets are non-refundable.
- Sorry, there are no tickets available.
- Would you like to make a reservation for another night?
- I would like two seats for tonight's performance, please.
- Where are the best seats you have left?
- Do you have anything in the first four rows?
- Do you have matinees?
- How much are the tickets?
- Is it possible to exchange these for another night?
- Do you take a check/credit cards?
- How long does the show run? About two hours.
- When does the show close?
- Is there an intermission? There is an intermission.
- Where are the rest rooms?
- Where is the cloakroom?
- Is there anywhere we can leave our coats?
- Do you sell concessions?
- How soon does the curtain go up?
- Did you make a reservation?
- What name did you reserve the tickets under?
- The usher will give you your programme.

At the Drugstore (*UK* Chemist)

- Prescription, tablet, pill, cream, suppository, laxative, sedative, injection, bandage, sticking plasters, cotton wool, gauze, alcohol, thermometer, sanitary towels, napkins, toothpaste, toothbrush, paper tissues, duty chemist.
- Fever, cold, cough, headache, toothache, diarrhea, constipation, sickness, insomnia, sunburn, insect bite.
- I am looking for something for ...
- Could you give me ...?
- Could you give me something for ...?
- I need some aspirin/antiseptic/eye drops/foot powder.
- I need razor blades and shaving foam.
- What are the side effects of this drug?
- Will this make me drowsy?
- Should I take this with meals?

At the Cosmetics Counter

- Soap, shampoo, deodorant, shower gel, hair spray, sun tan cream, comb, hairbrush, toothpaste, toothbrush, make up, cologne water, lipstick, perfume, hair remover, scissors, face lotion, cleansing cream, razor, shaving foam.

At the Bookshop/Newsagent's

- I would like to buy a book on the history of the city.
- Has this book been translated into Japanese?
- Have you got Swedish newspapers/magazines/books?
- Where can I buy a road map?

At the Photography Shop

- I want a 36 exposure film for this camera.
- I want new batteries for my camera.
- Could you develop this film?
- Could you develop this film with two prints of each photograph?
- How much does developing cost?
- When will the photographs be ready?
- My camera is not working, would you have a look at it?
- Do you take passport (ID) photographs?
- I want an enlargement of this one and two copies of this other.
- Have you got a 64-megabyte data card to fit this camera?
- How much would a 128-megabyte card be?
- How many megapixels is this one?
- Has it got an optical zoom?
- Can you print the pictures on this CD?

At the Florist

- I would like to order a bouquet of roses.
- You can choose violets and orchids in several colors.
- Which flowers are the freshest?
- What are these flowers called?
- Do you deliver?
- Could you please send this bouquet to the NH Abascal hotel manager at 47 Abascal St. before noon?
- Could you please send this card too?

Paying

- Where is the cash machine?
- Is there a cashpoint near here?
- How much is that all together?
- Will you pay cash or by credit card?
- Next in line (queue).
- Could you gift-wrap it for me?
- Can I have a receipt, please?
- Is there a cashpoint near here?
- Can I have a receipt, please?

At the Hairdresser

When I was in Boston I went to a hairdresser's and my lack of fluency was responsible for a drastic change in my image for a couple of months so that my wife almost did not recognize me when I picked her up at Logan on one of her multiple visits to New England. I can assure you that I will never forget the word "sideburns"; the hairdresser, a robust Afro-American lady, drastically cut them before I could recall the name of this insignificant part of my facial hair. To tell you the truth, I did not know how important sideburns were until I didn't have them.

If you do not trust an unknown hairdresser, "just a trim" would be a polite way of avoiding a disaster.

I recommend, before going to the hairdresser, a thorough review of your guide so that you get familiar with key words such as: scissors, comb, brush, dryer, shampooing, hair style, hair cut, manicure, dyeing, shave, beard, moustache, sideburns (!) (US), (sideboards (UK)), fringe, curl or plait.

Men and Women

- How long will I have to wait?
- Is the water OK? It is fine/too hot/too cold.
- My hair is greasy/dry.
- I have dandruff.
- I am losing a lot of hair.
- A shampoo and rinse, please.
- How would you like it?
- Are you going for a particular look?
- I want a (hair) cut like this.
- Just a trim, please.
- However you want.
- Is it OK?
- That's fine, thank you.

- How much is it?
- How much do I owe you?
- Do you do highlights?
- I would like a tint, please.

Men

- I want a shave.
- A razor cut, please.
- Just a trim, please.
- Leave the sideburns as they are (!) (*UK* sideboards).
- Trim the moustache.
- Trim my beard and moustache, please.
- Towards the back, without any parting.
- I part my hair on the left/in the middle.
- Leave it long.
- Could you take a little more off the top/the back/the sides?
- How much do you want me to take off?

Women

- How do I set your hair?
- What hair style do you want?
- I would like my hair dyed.
- Same color?
- A little darker/lighter.
- I would like to have a perm (permanent wave).

Cars

As always, begin with key words. Clutch, brake, blinkers (*UK* indicators), trunk (*UK* boot), tank, gearbox, windshield (*UK* windscreen) wipers, (steering) wheel, unleaded gas (*UK* petrol), etc, must belong to your fund of knowledge of English, as well as several usual sentences such as:
- How far is the nearest gas (petrol) station? 20 miles from here.
- In what direction? Northeast/Los Angeles.

At the Gas/Petrol Station

- Fill it up, please.
- Unleaded, please.
- Could you top up the battery, please?
- Could you check the oil, please?

- Could you check the tyre pressures, please?
- Do you want me to check the spare tyre too? Yes, please.
- Pump number 5, please.
- Can I have a receipt, please.

At the Garage

- My car has broken down.
- What do you think is wrong with it?
- Can you mend a puncture?
- Can you take the car in tow to downtown Boston?
- I see ..., kill the engine, please.
- Start the engine, please.
- The car goes to the right and overheats.
- Have you noticed if it loses water/gas/oil?
- Yes, it's losing oil.
- Does it lose speed?
- Yes, and it doesn't start properly.
- I can't get it into reverse.
- The engine makes funny noises.
- Please, repair it as soon as possible.
- I wonder if you can fix it temporarily.
- How long will it take to repair?
- I am afraid we have to send for spare parts.
- The car is very heavy on petrol.
- I think the right front tyre needs changing.
- I guess the valve is broken.
- Is my car ready?
- Have you finished fixing the car?
- Did you fix the car?
- Do you think you can fix it today?
- Could you mend a puncture?
- I think I've got a puncture rear offside.
- The spare's flat as well.
- I've run out of petrol.

At the Car Park

- Do you know where the nearest car park is?
- Are there any free spaces?
- How much is it per hour?
- Is the car park supervised?
- How long can I leave the car here?

Renting a Car

- I want to rent a car.
- I want to hire a car.
- For how many days?
- Unlimited mileage?
- What is the cost per mile?
- Is insurance included?
- You need to leave a deposit.

How Can I Get To ...?

- How far is Minneapolis?
- It is not far. About 12 miles from here.
- Is the road good?
- It is not bad, although a bit slow.
- Is there a toll road between here and Berlin?
- How long does it take to get to Key West?
- I am lost. Could you tell me how I can get back to the toll road.

Having a Drink (or Two)

Nothing is more desirable than a drink after a hard day of meetings. In such a relaxed situation embarrassing incidents can happen. Often, there is a difficult counter-question to a simple "Can I have a beer?" such as "would you prefer lager?" or "small, medium or large, sir?" From my own experience, when I was a beginner, I hated counter-questions and I remember my face flushing when in a pub in London, instead of giving me the beer I asked for, the barman responded with the entire list of beers in the pub. "I have changed my mind, I'll have a Coke instead" was my response to both the "aggression" I suffered from the barman and the embarrassment resulting from my lack of fluency. "We don't serve Coke here, sir." These situations can spoil the most promising evening so ... let's review a bunch of usual sentences:

- Two beers please, my friend will pay.
- Two pints of bitter and half a lager, please.
- Where can I find a good place to go for a drink?
- Where can we go for a drink at this time of the evening?
- Do you know any pubs with live music?
- What can I get you?
- I'm driving. Just an orange juice, please.
- A glass of wine and two beers, please.

- A gin and tonic.
- A glass of brandy. Would you please warm the glass?
- Scotch, please.
- Do you want it plain, with water, or on the rocks?
- Make it a double.
- I'll have the same again, please.
- Two cubes of ice and a teaspoon, please.
- This is on me.
- What those ladies are having is on me.

On the Phone

Many problems start when you lift the receiver. You hear a continuous purring different from the one you are used to in your country or a strange sequence of rapid pips. Immediately "what the hell am I supposed to do right now" comes to your mind, and we face one of the most embarrassing situations for non-fluent speakers. The phone has two added difficulties: firstly, its immediacy and, secondly, the absence of image ("if I could see this guy I would understand what he was saying"). Do not worry, the preliminary exchanges in this conversational scenario are few. Answering machines are another different, and tougher, problem and are out of the scope of this survival guide. Just a tip: do not hang up. Try to catch what the machine is saying and give it another try in case you are not able to follow its instructions. Many doctors, as soon as they hear the unmistakable sound of these devices, terrified, hang up thinking they are too much for them. Most messages are much easier to understand and less mechanical than those given by "human" (and usually bored) operators.

- Where are the public phones, please?
- Where is the nearest call-box?
- This telephone is out of order.
- Operator, what do I dial for the USA?
- Hold on a moment ... number one.
- Would you get me this number please?
- Dial straight through.
- What time does the cheap rate begin?
- Have you got any phone cards, please?
- Can I use your cell/mobile phone, please?
- Do you have a phone book (directory)?
- I'd like to make a reverse charge call to Korea.
- I am trying to use my phone card, but I am not getting through.
- Hello, this is Dr. Vida speaking.
- The line is engaged.
- There's no answer.

- It's a bad line.
- I've been cut off.
- I would like the number for Dr. Vida on Green Street.
- What is the area code for Los Angeles?
- I can't get through to this number. Would you dial it for me?
- Can you put me through to Spain?

Emergency Situations

- I want to report a fire/a robbery/an accident.
- This is an emergency. We need an ambulance/the police.
- Get me the police and hurry.

In the Bank

Nowadays, the spread of credit cards makes this section virtually unnecessary but, in my experience, when things go really wrong you may need to go to a bank. Fluency disappears in stressful situations so, in case you have to solve a bank problem, review not only this bunch of sentences but the entire section in your guide.

- Where can I change money?
- I'd like to change 200 Euros.
- I want to change 1000 Euros into Dollars/Pounds.
- Could I have it in tens, please?
- What's the exchange rate?
- What's the rate of exchange from Euros to Dollars?
- What are the banking hours?
- I want to change this travelers' check.
- Have you received a transfer from Rosario Nadal addressed to Fiona Shaw?
- Can I cash this bearer check?
- I want to cash this check.
- Do I need my ID to cash this bearer check?
- Go to the cash desk.
- Go to counter number 5.
- May I open a current account?
- Where is the nearest cash machine?
- I am afraid you don't seem to be able to solve my problem. Can I see the manager?
- Who is in charge?
- Could you call my bank in France? There must have been a problem with a transfer addressed to myself.

At the Police Station

- Where is the nearest police station?
- I have come to report a ...
- My wallet has been stolen.
- Can I call my lawyer (*UK* solicitor)?
- I have been assaulted.
- My laptop has disappeared from my room.
- I have lost my passport.
- I will not say anything until I have spoken to my lawyer/solicitor.
- I have had a car accident.
- Why have you arrested me? I've done nothing.
- Am I under caution?
- I would like to call my embassy/consulate.